Learning to Lead in
PHYSICAL THERAPY

Learning to Lead in
PHYSICAL THERAPY

Editor
Jennifer Green-Wilson, PT, MBA, EdD
Assistant Professor
SUNY Brockport
Brockport, New York
Principal
Institute for Business Literacy and Leadership
Rochester, New York

Associate Editor
Stacey Zeigler, PT, DPT, MS
Clinical Professor
Clarkson University
Owner
Fun in Aging Physical Therapy, PC
Potsdam, New York

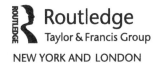

Routledge
Taylor & Francis Group

NEW YORK AND LONDON

Learning to Lead in Physical Therapy Instructor's Manual is available. Don't miss this important companion to *Learning to Lead in Physical Therapy*. To obtain the *Instructor's Manual*, please visit http://www.routledge.com/9781630916589

Cover Artist: Lori Shields

First published in 2020 by SLACK Incorporated

Published 2024 by Routledge
605 Third Avenue, New York, NY 10158

and by Routledge
4 Park Square, Milton Park, Abingdon, Oxon OX14 4RN

Routledge is an imprint of the Taylor & Francis Group, an informa business

© 2020 Taylor & Francis Group

Library of Congress Cataloging-in-Publication Data

Names: Green-Wilson, Jennifer, editor. | Zeigler, Stacey, editor.
Title: Learning to lead in physical therapy / editor, Jennifer Green-Wilson
    ; associate editor, Stacey Zeigler.
Description: Thorofare, NJ : SLACK Incorporated, [2020] | Includes
    bibliographical references and index.
Identifiers: LCCN 2020015263 (print) | ISBN 9781630916589 (hardcover)
Subjects: MESH: Leadership | Physical Therapists
Classification: LCC RM725 (print) | NLM WB 460 | DDC
    615.8/2--dc23
LC record available at https://lccn.loc.gov/2020015263

ISBN: 9781630916589 (pbk)
ISBN: 9781003524816 (ebk)

DOI: 10.4324/9781003524816

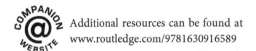
Additional resources can be found at
www.routledge.com/9781630916589

DEDICATION

To my mentors—the Rev. Susan Shafer, Dr. Dianne Cooney-Miner, Dr. Barbara A. Tschoepe, Dr. Diane Clark, and Angie Phillips—for believing in me and supporting me from start to finish. To my children—Ericka, Jessie, and Jeremy—for your love; for cheering me on; for taking away my cell phone; for grocery shopping, cleaning the house, and doing yardwork; and for keeping me focused on the "light at the end of the *long* tunnel." To my dogs—Ellison, Machia, and Gracie—for being close, hour after hour after hour. To Mario—for your heart and patience. To my dear friend and colleague—Dr. Stacey Zeigler—a huge thank you for your *unlimited* passion; for our writing retreats, especially near the water; for the endless fun stuff and snacks; for our road trips; and for all the telephone calls and Skype and Zoom check-ins. To my mom and dad—Mary Lou and A. Wesley Green—a heartfelt thank you for your love and support. To my dad—even though you are not here, please know that I keep your quiet sense of humor close at heart, especially when goals seem impossible.

Jennifer Green-Wilson, PT, MBA, EdD

I would like to dedicate this book:
- To Mom, Dad, Grandma, and Nana, who taught me the value of tenacity, hard work, and caring.
- To Samuel B. Feitelberg, whose leadership has been an inspiration.
- To my students, who are changing the world with their leadership.
- To my patients and clients, who challenge and inspire me to keep on leading.

Stacey Zeigler, PT, DPT, MS

CONTENTS

ACKNOWLEDGMENTS

The editors would like to express their sincere appreciation to the following individuals and contributors:

- Z. Annette Iglarsh and Barbara A. Tschoepe—thank you for providing the friendship, confidence, and mentorship for igniting the start of our dream to publish a textbook on leadership.

- Contributing authors—thank you for your continued patience, dedication, and knowledge in developing the content of this first edition.

- Authors of the forewords, leadership vignettes, and case studies—thank you for sharing your personal stories of your own leadership journeys. These have enriched our messages and demonstrated models for others to follow as they develop their own leadership capacity.

- Geneva Richard Johnson—thank you for role-modeling tenacity and inspiring innovation in physical therapy education.

- Sheila Nicholson—thank you for sharing your passion for leadership. Your transformational legacy will live on in our hearts, and we will miss you.

- Doctor of physical therapy programs with a vision for leadership—thank you to the University of Alabama at Birmingham, the University of Vermont, Clarkson University, Mary Baldwin University, Misericordia University, Regis University, and the University of Incarnate Word for their willingness to be early adopters for integrating personal leadership.

- HPA The Catalyst LAMP Institute for Leadership—we deeply appreciate the opportunity that the LAMP Institute for Leadership provided in helping us to start the fly wheel of leadership development in physical therapy. As a catalyst, you have challenged us to explore, discover, and inspire our own personal leadership journeys.

ABOUT THE EDITORS

Jennifer Green-Wilson, PT, MBA, EdD is an Assistant Professor in the Department of Health Care Studies at SUNY Brockport in New York. She is also the principal of the Institute for Business Literacy and Leadership (also known as the Leadership Institute). She is the former Director of the Institute for Leadership in Physical Therapy (LAMP) for HPA The Catalyst of the American Physical Therapy Association (APTA), and former member of the APTA Private Practice Section Education Committee. She served as a Director on the Board of Directors of the APTA from 2011 to 2014. Dr. Green-Wilson speaks nationally and internationally on topics related to leadership, business literacy, and management in health care; has been invited to submit short articles for APTA's "Business Sense" section of *PT in Motion*; and was awarded a national research grant from the HPA Section in 2009. Additionally, she was awarded HPA The Catalyst's LAMPLighter Leadership Award in February 2014, the Rochester Hearing and Speech Center's James DeCaro Leadership Award in 2017, and the Physical Therapy Association of Georgia's R. M. Barney Poole Leadership Academy Award for Excellence in Leadership and Education in 2019.

Dr. Green-Wilson works with doctor of physical therapy programs and diverse health care organizations across the country, helping strengthen the development of practice management, business literacy, and leadership skills at entry-level and in contemporary practice. Dr. Green-Wilson holds an EdD degree in executive leadership from St. John Fisher College in Rochester, New York; an MBA from the Rochester Institute of Technology; and a BS in physical therapy from Queen's University in Kingston in Ontario, Canada.

Stacey Zeigler, PT, DPT, MS is a Clinical Professor in the Department of Physical Therapy at Clarkson University in Potsdam, New York. She is also the founder and owner of Fun in Aging Physical Therapy, PC, a physical therapy private practice focusing on in-home wellness and fitness for older adults. She has been a faculty member for HPA The Catalyst of the APTA LAMP programs since 2001, and has held elected and volunteer positions at the district, chapter, and national levels of the APTA. She speaks nationally and internationally on topics related to leadership, patient autonomy, and health promotion with an emphasis on the application of these topics to the clinical practice of physical therapists. Dr. Zeigler was awarded HPA The Catalyst's LAMPLighter Leadership Award in February 2016, Jefferson Community College's Distinguished Alumni Professional Achievement Award in 2013, HPA The Catalyst's Outstanding Service Award in 2012, and the Dr. Marilyn Moffat Distinguished Service Award from the New York Physical Therapy Association in 2011.

Dr. Zeigler has held formal and informal leadership roles within and outside of the profession of physical therapy and currently focuses her efforts on inspiring the leaders of tomorrow at the grassroots level through education and mentorship. Dr. Zeigler earned her DPT from Simmons College, Boston, Massachusetts, in 2005, an MS in community health administration and wellness promotion from California College for Health Sciences, National City, California, in 2001, and a BS in physical therapy from Upstate Medical University, Syracuse, New York, in 1994.

Contributing Authors

Eileen C. Bach, PT, DPT, MEd
 (Chapter 7 Leadership Vignette)
New York, New York

Janet R. Bezner, PT, DPT, PhD, FAPTA
 (Chapter 1 Case Study)
National Board Certified Health &
 Wellness Coach
Associate Professor
Department of Physical Therapy
Texas State University
Round Rock, Texas

Jill Black, PT, DPT, EdD (Chapter 7)
Associate Dean and Associate Professor
Institute for Physical Therapy Education
Widener University
Chester, Pennsylvania

Diane E. Clark, PT, DScPT, MBA
 (Chapter 9 Leadership Vignette)
Associate Professor Emerita
The University of Alabama at Birmingham
Birmingham, Alabama

Beth Danehy, MA, MS, LMFT, CEAP
 (Chapter 8)
Director
Faculty & Employee Assistance Program
University of Virginia
Charlottesville, Virginia

Joshua D'Angelo, PT, DPT
 (Chapter 11 Case Study)
Board Certified Specialist in Orthopedics
CEO, President, and Co-Founder
 MovementX
COO, Vice President, and Co-Founder
Move Together
Co-Founder
PT Day of Service
Adjunct Professor
The George Washington University
Arlington, Virginia

Efosa L. Guobadia, DPT
 (Chapter 11 Case Study)
CEO of the Collective
FFITT Health
Move Together
PT Day of Service
PT Haven
Baldwin, New York

Karen M. Hughes, PT, MS, LSS BB
 (Chapter 6 Leadership Vignette)
Vice President
HPA The Catalyst Section of the
 American Physical Therapy Association
Buffalo, New York

Richard Jackson, PT, OCS (Chapter 11
 Leadership Vignette)
The Jackson Clinics, LP
The Jackson Clinics Foundation, Inc
Middleburg, Virginia

Geneva Richard Johnson, PhD, DPT (Hon),
 FAPTA (Foreword)
Physical Therapy Educational Consultant
Editor, Darbonne and Bartolett Publishers
Baton Rouge, Louisiana

Nancy R. Kirsch, PT, DPT, PhD, FAPTA
 (Chapter 10)
Vice Chair
Rehabilitation and Movement Sciences
Rutgers, The State University of New Jersey
Newark, New Jersey

Craig Moore, PT, MS, MBA
 (Chapter 3 Leadership Vignette)
AdventHealth
Orlando, Florida

Karen Mueller, PT, DPT, PhD
 (Chapter 5 Leadership Vignette)
Professor
Department of Physical Therapy and
 Athletic Training
Northern Arizona University
Flagstaff, Arizona

Sheila K. Nicholson, PT, DPT, JD, MBA, MA (Chapter 8 Leadership Vignette)
Lithia, Florida

Angela M. Phillips, PT (Chapter 4 Leadership Vignette)
President and CEO
Images and Associates
McKinney, Texas

Emma K. Stokes, BSc (Physio), MSc, MSc Mgmt, PhD (Chapter 1 Leadership Vignette)
Associate Professor and Department Head
Physiotherapy & Rehabilitation Science
Qatar University
Doha, Qatar
President
World Physiotherapy

Laura Lee (Dolly) Swisher, PT, MDiv, PhD, FAPTA (Chapter 10 Leadership Vignette)
Professor
School of Physical Therapy & Rehabilitation Sciences
USF Health Morsani College of Medicine
University of South Florida
Tampa, Florida

Barbara A. Tschoepe, PT, DPT, PhD, FAPTA (Chapter 11)
Catherine Worthingham Fellow
Education Consultant
Rise to the Top Consulting
Boulder, Colorado

Jerre van den Bent, PT (Chapter 2 Leadership Vignette)
Founder and CEO
THERAPY 2000
Dallas, Texas

Beth Whitehead, PT, MPH (Foreword)
Founder, Owner, and CEO
HealthActions, PA
Jackson, Alabama

PREFACE

I learned about transformational leadership while working with physical therapist students over a 5-year period from 2004 to 2008. Here is my story.

I started teaching in a physical therapy program in upstate New York as an adjunct faculty in 1999. I discovered that I loved teaching physical therapist students, but quickly realized that many perceive the content areas in which I am most passionate as nonclinical. Specifically, I love to help students learn about the business of physical therapist practice, health policy, health systems, payment, professional issues, developing interpersonal skills, leadership, and effective teamwork. Therefore, for many years, I worked intentionally to facilitate learning experiences that are relevant and applied to help students integrate these critical nonclinical skills and knowledge into clinical practice, and to help them understand that they have many roles to fulfill as physical therapists in contemporary practice.

Then, one day in 2003, the Chair of the physical therapy program assigned me the task of starting an on-campus physical therapy clinic to serve the underserved. I still remember this day of "hallway delegation." I also remember the next day when I left the pool after a good swim with my new "swim revelation": the students would be responsible for starting the physical therapy clinic—not me! I redesigned the Business of Physical Therapy course and, for 5 years, in my role as the Faculty Coach (aka Course Coordinator), the students started and expanded the clinic while learning about real-world marketing, operations management, financial management and fundraising, teamwork, and the importance of leadership in driving change and successful clinical practice. Students reported that this opportunity to experience the dual roles of being the clinician and the practice/business manager at the same time during the same semester had become one of their most valuable learning experiences in preparing them as physical therapists for clinical practice.

What was truly exciting for me was that each year, for 5 consecutive years, I had a new cohort of physical therapist students in my "leadership lab" in which I had to lead—to mentor and guide them in developing their understanding of the business side of physical therapist practice, practicing their management and leadership skills, working effectively in teams, and navigating conflict and multiple stakeholders invested in the clinic's success. So began my discovery of the power of transformational leadership. **I learned about transformational leadership from working with physical therapist students!** I discovered that when I valued the students and their potential to lead, they led as empowered, engaged, and passionate followers. They inspired me; I inspired them. Together, we all grew. Together, we delivered amazing outcomes; a win-win-win learning experience for all—especially for our patients and clients and their families.

In 2008, I started my doctorate in education in executive leadership at St. John Fisher College in Rochester, New York. Concurrently, I assumed the role as Director for HPA The Catalyst's (American Physical Therapy Association) Leadership, Administration, Management, and Professionalism/Practice program, and was charged by HPA's Board of Directors to launch the new beginning of the program's Institute for Leadership in Physical Therapy. What a wonderful opportunity! Imagine how much fun it was to study formally about leadership, after spending the past 5 years teaching and mentoring physical therapist students about leadership, while developing an experiential, evidence-based curricular model for leadership development for physical therapists across the United States!

I have written this textbook because I have witnessed firsthand our potential as physical therapists—at all levels in clinical practice—to be leaders within the health care system and within our communities in the United States and, hopefully, beyond. Change requires leadership, and we work within an industry that has been and will continue to experience rapid and sometimes chaotic change. Unfortunately, developing leadership skills during entry-level preparation and post-professionally has not been a priority in many physical therapist programs and practices. I hope that by writing this textbook, we can help change our focus by realizing the immediate need and vital opportunity we have to build our leadership capacity as a profession— for tomorrow, and for our future.

Audience

The ideal audience for this textbook is *everyone* in physical therapist practice—formal and informal leaders. My hope is that this textbook helps physical therapist students, academic faculty, clinical faculty, and clinicians learn to lead by becoming personal leaders at all levels and in all areas of practice, education, and research within the profession of physical therapy and within health care teams. I also hope that this resource helps physical therapist assistants—as students and as practitioners—so that we may strengthen our collective ability to leverage high-performing teams and to collaborate better on interprofessional teams.

Approach

There are many resources, models, and frameworks available that connect directly and indirectly to leadership and leadership development. In addition, new conversations and resources are emerging all the time, especially related to the urgent need for leadership development within health care. As a team of co-authors, we decided to compile and integrate many existing and emerging evidence-based, useful, and relevant frameworks together to expose you to:

- The need for leadership development within physical therapy
- The concept of personal (informal) leadership
- Critical topics related to the process of learning to lead
- Models and frameworks used outside and within the health care industry
- How you can assess and start to develop your own leadership capacity
- How you can progress your development over time

I have integrated and shared *My Vision of Leadership* throughout this textbook. This vision reflects many of my core beliefs and strategies that I use as a leader every day in practice—regardless of my role:

- Leadership is about building relationships with people, and through those relationships, great things can happen.
- Everyone on the team can add value, and it is important to include each person's contribution in some way.
- A leader inspires each person to want to contribute.
- A leader guides the journey but does not dictate the path.
- Leadership is about adapting to the situation without compromising the vision.
- Leadership is about leveraging failures to foster deep learning.
- Great leadership is empowering ("powerful") and energizing.
- Great leadership can be threatening.

Organization

We have divided this textbook into 3 distinct units or conversations to help individuals learn how to lead to become personal leaders and to build their own leadership capacity as physical therapists. Unit 1, which includes Chapters 1 through 4, is focused on helping students, faculty, and clinicians gain knowledge about personal leadership and start to develop their own personal leadership skills from inside-out. I like to call this stage of leadership development as the stage in which individuals "hold up their own mirrors" to develop greater self-awareness and a better understanding of their own core—their values, passions, and beliefs that are needed to fuel their ability to demonstrate effective leadership behaviors. We use evidence-based models and frameworks to help individuals start to understand effective and ineffective leadership styles and to learn how to self-manage, develop, and adapt their own authentic "leadership styles" in various situations.

In Unit 2, covering content presented in Chapters 5 through 8, we build on the fundamental knowledge and skills presented in Unit 1 to help individuals start to apply different leadership skills in specific situations. By doing so, individuals who are learning to lead can develop greater leadership effectiveness while working with other people.

In Unit 3, Chapters 9 through 11, we start to address how individuals who are learning to lead can start to lead others intentionally in formal and informal leadership situations and roles.

An Instructor's Manual is available as an additional resource to guide the process of teaching how to learn to lead OR learning to lead.

Jennifer Green-Wilson, PT, MBA, EdD

Foreword:
Leadership in Physical Therapy

Physical therapy is a health care profession shrouded in the midst of an uncertain future. Declaration of what that future will be remains open to physical therapists who are the practitioners in this age of uncertainty, but cannot be delayed indefinitely without undesirable consequences.

The future of physical therapy is in our hands and hearts, if we choose to take actions directed by our heads. We face obstacles that may seem insurmountable, but the path to success is provided in this wonderfully timely text. The authors explain why leadership by all of us is critical to our survival as a profession. They challenge us to be "leaders in this cause" and to educate present and future learners in the profession to accept their responsibilities as leaders. Choosing employment environments following graduation is important to their development as leaders of the future.

Physical therapy has been evolving as a profession since World War I with the appointment of women as reconstruction aides (1918). After discharge from the United States Army, they declared themselves to be "physiotherapists"—a designation used in England and other European nations. Fortunately, this group decided to found the American Physiotherapy Association with 21 members (now numbering more than 95,000). They organized programs in hospitals to "train" others as physiotherapists. Our first leaders were women who accepted the responsibilities inherent in the designation of "leader."

Today we must follow their legacy as we face the necessity of educating all practitioners as leaders because:

- We are known now by the public we serve as competent health care practitioners. However, as licensed professionals, we cannot provide our services universally without restrictions.
- We are still required by legislation in some states to have a referral from a physician or other licensed practitioner before initiating physical therapy beyond an evaluation.
- Payment for the delivery of physical therapy services can be denied without "a prescription from a physician." Leaders are needed to change the laws that restrain us.
- External controls hamper our ability to serve many who could benefit from the guidance and services of a physical therapist in a community environment.
- Physical therapists are educated now to provide services as primary health care practitioners.
- Physical therapy as a profession has 3 outstanding components: the delivery of physical therapy services (directly to individuals and groups), education, and research. Those components cannot be divided in practice, because no one can be effective without the other 2 in place.
- Leadership is essential in affirming the freedom to practice as Doctors of Physical Therapy (DPTs), all of whom are graduates of an institution accredited by the Commission on Accreditation in Physical Therapy Education (CAPTE).
- Physical therapy, like other health care professions, has broadened the scope of practice to include keeping people fit so they are able to function satisfactorily in society, and in employment environments, including academic environments as faculty.
- If physical therapy does not provide leaders to influence decision-makers about our role in primary health care—the future—we will be unable to practice as independent practitioners and will be restricted by rules others create for our practice.
- This is a crisis situation that is in need of strong leadership at all levels in clinical practice if we are to survive as a profession. Our leaders must be able to speak in tones of authority, ready to describe the knowledge, skills, and compassion we bring to our role as health care practitioners, and our intent to be accepted as equals with other health care practitioners in the United States and other nations.

The most important issue about leadership, I think, is that we are in crisis at all levels of decision-making. If we fail to take advantage of our opportunities to be at the table when decisions are being made, that will affect us and render us inadequate as leaders. Although we have improved over the years about dealing with issues that affect us, the intent to encourage attention to this crucial aspect of education is obvious in the book that Drs. Jennifer Green-Wilson, Stacey Zeigler, Barbara Tschoepe, and several of our colleagues have written. Emphasizing the critical role of leadership is an imperative inclusion in the curriculum.

Leadership Behaviors

Over the years, the watchwords for me have been these: passion, persistence, and patience. Other valuable behaviors are a vision of the consequences if action is delayed on an issue—small or large; prudence; generosity in sharing success; openness in acknowledging failures when those occur, sometimes beyond our control but real, nevertheless, and difficult to overcome; willingness to participate in projects that may not be one's highest priority at a given time; peacefulness in times of turmoil, especially those events beyond my control; and caution in assuming actions are designed to discredit any one person, especially me. My list of leadership behaviors includes kindness to peers, colleagues, patients and clients; receptivity to different approaches in care for the diagnosis of impaired function; readiness to learn new or different methods of solving problems; praise for others in the successful conclusion to a project or the handling of a difficult situation; honoring the contributions of peers and colleagues involved in the successful completion of a shared project; consistency in behavior; dependable and reliable in accepting responsibility for an assignment or a position as a leader. This not intended as an exhaustive list—many more behaviors describe a leader.

Leaders in any environment in the practice of physical therapy—that is, the delivery of physical services, education, and research—have identifiable behaviors. Some of those behaviors are listed below. Leaders are:

Accessible	Eager	Humble	Promoters	Thorough
Adaptable	Educated	Joyful	Proud	Thoughtful
Bold	Ethical	Kind	Receptive	Trustworthy
Caring	Forgiving	Knowledgeable	Responsible	Visionaries
Collaborators	Generous	Listeners	Responsive	Vivacious
Competent	Gentle	Mentors	Sensible	Zealous
Constant	Gracious	Open	Sensitive	Zestful
Dedicated	Helpful	Peaceful	Sharers	
Developers	Honest	Persistent	Tenacious	

As you read this special text written by Dr. Jennifer Green-Wilson and our colleagues, you may want to make additions to the list above. Their vision of the role of the physical therapist as leaders speaks with conviction to the necessity of incorporating in our curricula a strong emphasis on leadership as one of our most important functions. We could adopt the policy of "let not your light be unseen, but let it shine forth for all to see," so that our role in the evolving systems of health care cannot be ignored.

With the need for leaders to continue the advancement of physical therapy as a profession vital to health care, in this and other nations, all educational programs must accept responsibility for educating those leaders. This text is an inspiration to leaders and their successors.

Geneva Richard Johnson, PhD, DPT (Hon), FAPTA
Physical Therapy Educational Consultant
Editor, Darbonne and Bartolett Publishers
Baton Rouge, Louisiana

FOREWORD:
THE VALUE OF MENTORSHIP IN PHYSICAL THERAPY

The authors asked me to share some of my insights about Geneva R. Johnson, PhD, DPT (Hon), FAPTA, also known as Geanie, because of my personal friendship with her over the past 44 years. This is no small task, because she is a study in leadership, mentorship, and professionalism. Her contributions have spanned almost 70 years in APTA and beyond that as a physical therapist. She has influenced generations of physical therapists, directly and indirectly, during times of transition from the polio epidemic and aftermath of World War II, followed by times of change in educational requirements, until now. She attended every APTA conference from 1950 until 2019, when she decided it was becoming too difficult to travel. Her legacy of innovation in education and drive toward professionalism is celebrated every year at APTA's Education Leadership Conference (ELC) when the Physical Therapy Learning Institute (PTLI), a group she founded with Lynda Woodruff, PT, PhD, sponsors a keynote speaker to present The GRJ Forum for Innovations in Education to keep the drive for excellence alive.

A graduate of the University of Louisiana in Lafayette in 1942 in health and physical education and recreation, Geanie did not know she wanted to become a physical therapist, but this was a time when polio remained an epidemic and not long after the bombing of Pearl Harbor, so there was a real demand for physical therapists. She answered the call to service and completed the Army's certificate program in physical therapy at Lawson General Hospital in Atlanta in 1946.

While in the Army, in 1950 she married Bart Johnson, from Iowa, who was also serving in the military. As a devout Catholic, her greatest wish was to be the mother of about 10 children. When her prayers were not answered, she followed the call to become a leader in the physical therapy profession as the demand for physical therapists with more education increased.

In between many practice and administrative positions, Dr. Johnson completed her MA at the University of South Carolina in educational administration in 1959, and then her PhD in higher education from the University of Pittsburgh.

The drive for higher education in APTA began with Catherine Worthingham, PT, PhD, FAPTA, during the World War II years when polio was still an epidemic. President Roosevelt had created the National Foundation for Infantile Paralysis in 1928, and in 1938, it was named the March of Dimes. This greatly assisted fundraising to provide for research and education, which led to the development of the vaccines to eradicate the disease in this country. It also contributed to education, particularly for physical therapists. Dr. Worthingham served as the Director for Professional Education for the Foundation, and was able to direct funding for educational preparation. In the late 1950s, she chose Case Western Reserve University (CWRU) to receive funding to develop a postgraduate entry-level physical therapy degree. Dr. Johnson was recruited to consult for that program and serve as an Assistant Professor. The Director of the program became ill during the early years, and Dr. Johnson was recruited to become an Associate Professor and Director of the Physical Therapy School in 1964. In 1967, she and her associate, Dorothy Pinkston, PT, PhD, FAPTA, proposed a transitional doctorate degree, but it failed to be funded during a challenging economic time throughout the time of the Vietnam War. Funding for physical therapy was not impacted, but funding for other educational programs like medicine were, so monies were directed to maintain the medical school.

Dr. Johnson moved back to Houston and accepted a position with Baylor University, where she had been the Coordinator of Services from 1954 to 1957. She became the Director for Texas Institute for Rehabilitation and Research, where she remained until 1984 when she became a full-time consultant in higher education.

My introduction to Dr. Johnson came in 1975 when I attended my first APTA conference as a relatively new graduate from University of Alabama at Birmingham (UAB). My program director and mentor at UAB, Marilyn Gossman, PT, PhD, FAPTA, was a graduate of CWRU and Dr. Johnson was her mentor. Marilyn was running for the APTA Board of Directors that year and needed someone to "look after" Dr. Johnson during an event because she was unable to spend much time with her. I knew Marilyn meant for me to get her a glass of wine, food and chat with her, but the assignment began a lifetime of friendship and mentorship.

Dr. Johnson has a deep passion for physical therapy and loves to talk about the future of the profession, and so do I. As one of those college graduates in 1970 who had limited access to physical therapy graduate school, I had been denied entrance to the Army's new post-graduate program in 1970 because I needed another year of prerequisites. I chose to go to UAB's baccalaureate entry-level program instead of waiting to reapply. I had already met Marilyn Gossman at UAB, and some of her faculty, who were also CWRU graduates. I trusted that was the best option for me, since my mother had become ill, and I felt I needed to be closer to home.

Dr. Johnson and I shared other common experiences, like our educational background and her experiences at the William Beaumont Army Hospital in El Paso, Texas, where I had also done a pre-physical therapy internship. Both of us were serving as Directors of Physical Therapy Services; she was at the Texas Institute for Rehabilitation and Research, and I was at the Rotary Rehabilitation Center in Mobile, Alabama. Both facilities were involved in the care of spinal-cord-injured patients, and we both had interest in clinical research. I was completing a master's degree in public health and was working on a thesis for evaluating outcomes. In 1978, we were appointed to a task force by APTA's Section on Administration to study the characteristics of the Physical Therapy Administrator. It preceded the development of APTA's Health Policy and Administration Section's (HPA's) LAMP (Leadership, Administration, Management, Professionalism) as a continued educational opportunity for physical therapists.

Historically, UAB had already incorporated a lot of CWRU curriculum because Marilyn Gossman had become a Program Director before the age of 30 and had limited experience as a physical therapist or an educator. Dr. Johnson assisted Marilyn and her cohorts with development of the curriculum at UAB at the same time she and Dorothy Pinkston were developing the post-graduate doctorate curriculum for CWRU. Marilyn began to look at how to transition UAB to a post-graduate level, but met resistance from the Southern Dean's Association.

Marilyn Gossman, together with Geneva Johnson and many on APTA's Board of Directors, took up the campaign to transition all physical therapy programs to the post-graduate level. There was a strong proponent to keep the entry-level baccalaureate as the terminal degree, the master's for developing specialists, and the PhD to develop educators and researchers. However, studies showed that an undergraduate liberal arts education level prior to professional school developed a more well-rounded professional. In the APTA House of Delegates in 1979, Marilyn introduced RC14-79 to transition all physical therapy programs to the postgraduate level by 1990. I was serving in the House of Delegates, and it was a very momentous occasion. Dr. Johnson had planted a seed in Marilyn Gossman and nurtured it for years, and together a small group moved our profession forward—the way Mary McMillan did when she became the first President of the association, and the way Catherine Worthingham did when she focused on the future of physical therapy through education.

Geanie's Mary McMillan Lecture in 1985 called for the development of the professional doctorate. She said she expected to see it by 1990, and Creighton University opened the first professional doctorate in 1993. Geneva Johnson was the consultant who they asked whether they should begin with a doctorate or not, and it was reported that she "boldly" encouraged them to begin with the doctorate. She planted the seed, she nurtured it, and the leadership of the University followed her advice.

Geanie founded the Physical Therapy Learning Institute (PTLI) in 1991 to organize educational leaders to promote the transition to the professional doctorate, among other things. There was promotion of the problem-based learning model for professional education. In the late 90s, the Institute held a series of sessions in Atlanta to consider the physical therapist as a primary care practitioner. This remains an issue that is being studied, and she encourages us to continue that. She visualizes community primary care centers in rural, underserved areas that have doctors of nursing and doctors of physical therapy together working to improve health.

Dr. Johnson presented the Cerosoli lecture in 2008, and she called for schools to enlarge their enrollment and advised APTA's sections to become an Academy. APTA's geriatrics section became the first Academy in 2014. Others have since followed.

As a mentor to many, Geanie has been a visionary, a pioneer, an influencer, a challenger, a risk taker, and not a quitter. In 1995, at the age of 72, she implemented a problem-based curriculum in a master's program in a private university. A decline nationally in enrollment had a negative impact on the program, and it closed. However, at the age of 87, she answered an advertisement by a Catholic institution in San Antonio, Texas, who was seeking a Program Director for a developing physical therapy program. She and Bart took the train to San Antonio and met with the Chancellor of the University of Incarnate Word (UIW). She advised the Chancellor that she needed a school of physical therapy with a physical therapist as the dean. In 2012, the first school of physical therapy opened with its own Dean, Caroline Goulet, PT, PhD. The school incorporated a modified problem-based curriculum model.

Geanie is an excellent writer and communicator. I have read recommendations she has written for so many to receive awards, consultations she has done, and personal letters, but her greatest regret is never completing her book for academic administrators on leadership. Having these authors complete this particular book that develops leadership and mentorship throughout the profession of physical therapy is a source of joy for her, and she is happy for them and for our profession to have a better foundation to develop leadership at all levels.

I once shared a story with Geanie about the time I asked Marilyn Gossman if I could begin my second year of school a little late because I had the opportunity of a lifetime that conflicted with the start of school. Marilyn told me, "You will have to make that decision for yourself." I shared that I thought that was the first time someone had made me be responsible for making decisions for myself. It left an impression! Geanie laughed and said, "That is the same thing I told her."

Three of Dr. Johnson's favorite words are *passion*, *persistence*, and *professionalism*. She has certainly accomplished these in her life and more. She has influenced others to do the same. She seldom speaks of courage, but it is a quality that she has, and it has been the quality I have learned to appreciate more and more. Sometimes, when I have a challenge, I have a mental image of her being calm, poised, confident, and deliberate with her wording when she delivers a message that requires courage. I have not mastered her technique, but I am more mindful of when I need to have courage. Geanie plants seeds, and nurtures them as long as needed and beyond. Geanie prays for guidance, and she leads by example.

This is the value of mentorship. Pay it forward...

Beth Whitehead, PT, MPH
Founder, Owner, and CEO
HealthActions, PA
Jackson, Alabama

UNIT 1

LEADERSHIP AND
THOSE WHO LEAD

In the following 4 chapters of Unit 1, you will discover the first person that you lead is you! The term *personal leadership* will be used to describe this act of leading from the inside out—a self-driven style in which you are the facilitator of your own life. This approach requires personal autonomy and personal responsibility in choosing to act in specific ways to be, do, and think, so you can be the best version of yourself. Therefore, over the next 4 chapters, you will be asked to become more aware of who you are, who you want to be, how you tend to interact with others, how you influence action in the process of leading, and how you can develop a set of behaviors to become more effective at leading for results and change.

This unit is the vital foundation to the lessons in the remainder of the book. It is essential for you to start with the self in becoming the leader you want to be, and Unit 1 is designed to walk you through this process step by step. Welcome to Unit 1: Leadership and Those Who Lead.

At the Core of Leadership
Your Authentic Self

Jennifer Green-Wilson, PT, MBA, EdD
Stacey Zeigler, PT, DPT, MS

Authenticity is a collection of choices that we have to make every day. It's about the choice to show up and be real. The choice to be honest. The choice to let our true selves be seen.
— *Brené Brown, American scholar, author, and public speaker*

CHAPTER OBJECTIVES

➤ Describe the concept of leadership.
➤ Define *authentic leadership*.
➤ Discuss the characteristics needed for authentic leadership.
➤ Self-assess your leadership capacity.
➤ Self-assess your core values.
➤ Develop a personal mission statement.

Green-Wilson J, Zeigler S, eds.
Learning to Lead in Physical Therapy (pp 3-21).
© 2020 Taylor & Francis Group.

Leadership Vignette

Emma K. Stokes, BSc (Physio), MSc, MSc Mgmt, PhD

I am loyal when loyalty is earned and appropriate. In other words, I am not blindly loyal, and that relates to other core values of mine: integrity and fairness. I am committed to fairness and find it very hard to see others take actions that are unfair and driven by personal gain, rather than acting in the best interests of an organization, a project, or a cause. I value reliability and trustworthiness. I hope I have both, but recognize that I occasionally overcommit, and when this happens, it challenges other core values: doing my best, and working hard.

When I make a mistake, I try to learn from the error, and if I have hurt or upset someone, I apologize. I am forgiving and believe strongly in accepting I have been wrong and giving an unconditional apology. I don't find failure easy, but I am learning to learn from it. As Samuel Beckett wrote, "Ever try. Ever fail. No matter. Try again. Fail again. Fail better." When my sister and I made a mistake, Dad always said, "the person who made no mistakes, made nothing." It took me years to realize what this saying meant and that it was a key concept in helping me understand error is okay as long as you learn from it.

I am who I am, for better and worse. While I try to become more self-aware, recognizing the impact I have on others that can be both positive and negative, and while I try to learn more about how I can work better with others and lead, I do not try to change who I am as a person. I try to stay true to "me," and if that is not what organizations or groups want, then I review my options. I also step away from positions or activities when they challenge my moral compass on an ongoing basis.

Leadership requires many skills, knowledge, commitment, and passion. I have a deep commitment to and belief in physiotherapy as a profession, and this commitment and passion are strengths of mine to whatever I become involved in. The physiotherapists I have met around the world are passionate—some loudly, some quietly—and committed to helping their patients and the profession. This collective belief and commitment are powerful and can be leveraged more, I believe. I am very committed to supporting and developing the next generation of leaders—and my time with students and physiotherapists around the world convinces me that there is exceptional leadership potential in all of us.

LEADERSHIP CAPACITY: NATURE OR NURTURE?

Are the best leaders born (nature) or made (nurture)? The age-old debate about nature vs nurture can be applied to leadership and has resulted in a substantial body of literature (much of which will be referred to throughout this book). While qualities such as intelligence, problem-solving ability, and even being born to parents in leadership positions have been shown to give an individual a hereditary leg up for leadership, most of the characteristics and behaviors of effective leaders that you will read about in Chapters 2 and 3 of this book can be learned.

How do you go about learning to be a good leader? If you are reading this, you have already started your learning process. Realize also that you may have been developing certain skills of effective leaders (and possibly some ineffective ones) your entire life. In other words, you need to start to learn how to lead by learning more about yourself first. Then, you will understand more about why and where you need to go in your personal leadership development journey. While self-discovery is not always an easy task or a quick one, it is one that is worth the journey. This book is going to walk you through the entire process to becoming an effective leader. The first place to start is with you!

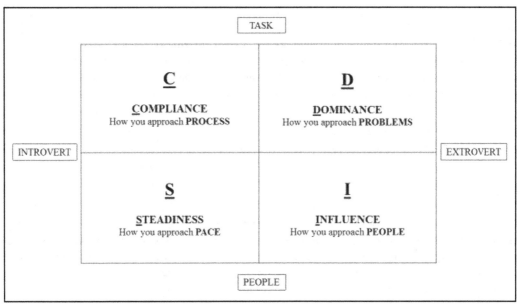

Figure 1-1. DISC Self-Assessment Framework. This self-assessment tool is useful to determine if you are more focused on the task or the people and relationships, and if you tend to be more of an extrovert or an introvert. It also helps you discover if you tend to be more forceful, direct, and results-oriented (D); more optimistic, fun, and talkative (I); steady, patient, and relaxed (S); or precise, accurate, and detail-oriented (C).

Natural Tendencies

What are your natural tendencies? Fortunately, or unfortunately, many factors of your personality are inherited. Qualities such as extroversion and sociability, which will be discussed later in this chapter, may run in your family and are considered traits of some of the most effective leaders. Have you ever caught yourself saying, "I sound just like my mother," or have you been told, "You act just like your father?" While some of these behaviors are inherited, others are learned. In fact, did you know that primary personality and behavioral styles are generally established by 7 years of age? What happens after this age is up to how each individual succumbs to nurture and intentional personal growth. A key concept in leading yourself and, ultimately, leading others is to be able to adapt your natural personality and behavioral tendencies to fit the needs of the situation and those around you. This is under your control—and definitely a learnable skill.

Activity 1-1: Discover Your Natural Personality Tendencies

Using self-assessment is highly recommended as one of the first steps to take in the process of discovering your authentic self. Two well-known, evidence-based self-assessments—the DISC[1] profile and the Myers-Briggs Type Indicator (MBTI)[2]—are described below.

- DISC[3] is a self-assessment tool used to improve work productivity, teamwork, and communica- tion (Figure 1-1). DISC helps you understand your personality, communication, and behavioral differences. The DISC profile (analysis) helps you to increase your individual self-awareness, determine what motivates you, identify what causes you stress, and demonstrate how you respond to conflict and how you solve problems. It also helps you learn how to adapt your own style, facilitate effective teamwork, and minimize team conflict.
- The MBTI[2] personality inventory helps you understand the ways in which you prefer to use your perception and judgment. After you decide on your preference in each category, you will be able to identify your own personality type, expressed as an acronym with 4 letters.

While the DISC[1] and the MBTI[2] are 2 of the most reliable industry standards, plenty of free inventories on the internet can also give you an acceptable start to understanding your natural tendencies and how they impact your interactions with others. A basic internet search for "personality test" or "colors personality profile" is a good starting point. Try taking one of these self-assessments, reflect, and then write what you learned about your personality tendencies.

_____

_____

_____

_____

Strengths

Strengths are expert skills, specific talents, or outstanding abilities. Strengths emerge when individuals exert deliberate practice, nurturing their strongest talents. Leaders who focus on leveraging strengths realize that great work emerges when people do what they love to do and when they are encouraged to apply their strengths in creative ways. Understanding your own strengths will help you determine your authentic self and define your passions for discussion later in this chapter.

Activity 1-2: Finding Your Strengths

CliftonStrengths[4] is the Gallup organization's proprietary, and very useful, assessment that helps discover your unique combination of strengths. For this activity, you will not need to access the complete tool. You can find descriptions of themes or strengths listed in the CliftonStrengths Theme Quick Reference Card available at https://www.strengthsquest.com/192458/clifton-strengths-theme-quick-reference-card.aspx.[5] From this list and from your general self-assessment, write down your strengths, then ask someone you know and trust to give you honest feedback about whether your list is perceived to be accurate.

_____	_____
_____	_____
_____	_____
_____	_____
_____	_____

Bottom Line!

Becoming a leader is a journey of reflection, self-learning, and practice. Nature, nurture, or otherwise, you must first develop an understanding of yourself, then take responsibility for your own development because the most difficult person you will ever have to lead is yourself.[6]

YOUR CONCEPT OF LEADERSHIP

Activity 1-3: What Does Leadership Mean to You?

Draw a picture of what leadership means to you (what image comes to mind when you think of leadership?):

Some view leadership as an arrangement of specific personality traits or characteristics, whereas others see leadership as encompassing certain skills, knowledge, behaviors, or competencies. What does your picture depict regarding your viewpoints of leadership?

Activity 1-4: A Leader's Impact

Describe a great leader you admire who displays leadership characteristics that you would like to emulate.

_____

_____

_____

_____

Leadership is viewed today as a dynamic process through which a person influences a group of individuals to achieve a shared goal, and as a trait that can be developed.[7,8] Leadership is about behavior—what leaders do—and effective leadership focuses on the relationship between those individuals who seek to lead and those who choose to follow,[9] with you being your very first follower. People expect leaders whom they admire to be honest, forward-looking, inspiring, competent, and intelligent.[9]

Do these characteristics match what you listed previously?

_____

_____

_____

How many of these characteristics do you feel already describe you?

_____

_____

_____

Bottom Line!

Becoming a leader requires work. Imagine the notion of holding up a mirror as the way to start your leadership journey. Leaders can only realize their unique and core passions, strengths, and values through a process of extensive self-examination that is intertwined with real-world experiences and ongoing reflection.[6,10,11] Therefore, who are you in relation to the leader you wish to become?

Figure 1-2. Dimensions of authentic leadership. This framework suggests that authentic leaders use 5 ways to display their authenticity. In this framework, authentic leaders work purposefully with passion, practice solid values, lead with heart, establish enduring relationships, and demonstrate self-discipline. (Reprinted with permission from George B, Sims P, Gergen, D. *True North: Discover Your Authentic Leadership.* San Francisco, CA: Jossey-Bass; 2007.)

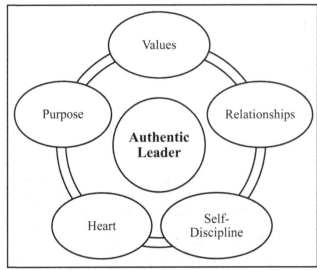

LEADERSHIP AND YOUR AUTHENTIC SELF

Authenticity, as it relates to leadership, is described as a necessary characteristic to be effective. Specifically, authentic leaders are genuine individuals; they bring a true sense of self to their leadership role—either as a formal or as an informal/personal leader. In other words, they know themselves from the inside-out. The following testimony by Janet Bezner, PT, DPT, PhD, FAPTA, Associate Professor, Department of Physical Therapy at Texas State University, emphasizes the need to experience this inside-out process to become authentic[12]:

> Several references identify that one of the most important characteristics of strong leadership is honesty, which is often used synonymously with authenticity. The ability to have self-awareness—to learn about yourself, change the behaviors that aren't serving you well, reflect on who you are as a leader—this is a prerequisite to being authentic. You can't be authentic if you don't know who you are, so authenticity and self-awareness are similar and very important to leadership. Followers deserve to know the truth, and authenticity helps people decide if they want to follow you. Authenticity provides the freedom to be who you are in every situation, to "walk the walk" and "talk the talk," and to harness the energy that is produced as a result of achieving a purpose above and beyond yourself.

As Dr. Bezner mentioned, authentic leaders demonstrate trustworthiness, honesty, and openness. They cultivate trust in such a way that it fosters relationships or genuine connections with others. Through these genuine connected relationships, energy, and engagement can be fueled.[11]

Authentic leaders use 5 ways to display their authenticity[6]:

1. Act purposefully with passion.
2. Practice solid values.
3. Lead with heart.
4. Establish enduring relationships.
5. Demonstrate self-discipline (Figure 1-2).[6]

The next section will take you through each of these 5 ways in further detail so that you can begin to understand more about your authentic self as you develop your personal leadership capacity.

Purpose With Passion

Purpose is the first display of authenticity. Finding the purpose of your leadership is a crucial starting point, and yet, this is something that is neither easy nor quick to accomplish. To gain purposeful self-awareness, authentic leaders must, at their core, understand themselves and their passions before they can find meaningful purpose in their leadership.[6] *Passion* can be described as an intense emotion—a compelling enthusiasm or desire for something. Passion is energy and that strong desire to do or share something that comes from within. Passion fuels everything; it motivates people and shapes the purpose behind personal and professional endeavors.[13] Leaders learning to lead will know that they are passionate about something when they become restless, when they wake up every morning driven to pursue their passions.[13]

A-HA! – DISCOVER YOUR PASSION

What makes you jump for joy, and why?

_____

What gives you energy?

_____

What motivates you?

_____

What inspires you?

_____

How does your passion influence your behaviors and decisions?

_____

_____

Passion can also be effectively expressed in the stories you share. Leaders use storytelling to move others to action, to stir emotions, and to connect with individuals on a personal level. A well-told story or narrative can inspire others and can influence an individual's perspective of different outcomes as well as build credibility and trust. Storytelling, or the language of leadership, will be discussed in more detail in Chapter 5, but you should think about and practice your own genuine stories as a way to help communicate your passions.

A-HA! – YOUR STORY

What is the story of you? What would you say if someone asked you, "So what's your story?"

_____

_____

_____

_____

_____

_____

What is a story about a struggle(s) or challenge(s) that you have faced and how you overcame it?

_____

_____

_____

_____

_____

_____

Summarize the answers you have just captured, and read your story out loud. Are you hearing your passions come through in your story? Do you hear yourself describing a crystal-clear sense of who you are, what you stand for, and how you got to this point in your life? If not, keep reading about the next 4 ways in which the authentic leader can display authenticity, as these will help you discover even more vital details about yourself. Then, you can use this additional information to come back to this activity to polish your story some more.

Solid Core Values

Developing yourself as a leader begins with knowing your convictions or values as well as your principles. *Principles* are rules or laws that are universal in nature, do not change over time, and transcend cultures and individuals. Examples of principles include fairness, integrity, and honesty. Individuals learning to lead can identify a set of principles to use as an internal compass. In this way, they can refer to these principles whenever they are unsure about a decision, need to set a boundary, or need to take a stand or evaluate an opportunity, behavior, or situation. Principles can help individuals determine their values.

Values are beliefs and opinions that individuals may hold regarding specific issues, situations, or ideas. Values are internal and subjective, and may change over time. Values are core, deeply foundational, and often emotional. Values are the innermost guiding principles that engage your passions and influence your decisions, commitments and responses towards others. Clarifying personal values helps individuals feel more motivated, creative, and committed. Being clear about personal values helps individuals learning to lead feel empowered, organized, and prepared for action.[9] Essentially, individuals must know what is sincerely important to them and why, as well as what is not important to them and why.

A-HA! – YOUR PRINCIPLES AND VALUES

Consider how your principles and values can be useful as you are learning to lead. For example, you can use your principles as a reference point to help you realize when your current values, goals, and behavior may be inconsistent or out of alignment. Because it is so critical to gain self-awareness of your principles and core values, take a few moments to answer the following questions:

What makes you who you are? What do you stand for and believe in, and why?

_____

_____

_____

_____

_____

_____

What are the universal, unchanging principles that you can clearly identify?

_____

_____

_____

_____

_____

_____

What are your most deeply held values, and why?

_____

_____

_____

_____

_____

_____

In what ways do your current behaviors reflect those values?

_____

_____

_____

_____

_____

_____

In what ways could your principles and core values guide your leadership?

_____

_____

_____

_____

_____

_____

The Rokeach Value Survey (RVS),[14] developed by social psychologist Milton Rokeach, is one of the most extensively used measures of human values. The RVS is a 36-item classification system or inventory consisting of 18 terminal values and 18 instrumental values.[14] *Terminal values* refer to desirable end-states of existence; these represent the goals that individuals would like to achieve. Interestingly, terminal values vary among different groups of people in different cultures. Examples of terminal values include a comfortable or prosperous life, a sense of accomplishment or of making lasting contributions, and free choice and independence.

TABLE 1-1. ROKEACH VALUE SURVEY SAMPLE		
SAMPLE TERMINAL VALUES	**RANKING OF TERMINAL VALUES**	**WHAT IS THE MEANING OF THIS VALUE TO YOU? WHY DOES IT MATTER?**
A comfortable life	1.	
An exciting life	2.	
Equality	3.	
Family security	4.	
Freedom	5.	
Health	6.	
Inner harmony	7.	
Mature love	8.	
National security	9.	
Social recognition	10.	
True friendship	11.	
Wisdom	12.	
A world of peace	13.	
Pleasure	14.	
Salvation	15.	
Self-respect	16.	
A sense of accomplishment	17.	
A world of beauty	18.	
		(continued)

Instrumental values refer to desirable modes of behavior or ways to achieve the terminal values. Instrumental values include ambition, hard work, aspiration, capability, competence and effectiveness, and honesty. Participants using the RVS are asked to organize the 18 terminal values, followed by the 18 instrumental values, into an order of importance to them. In this way, individuals start identifying their own guiding principles.

Activity 1-5: Explore Your Own Values

Use the Rokeach Value Survey sample (Table 1-1)[14] to start to assess your values. Put the following value in a priority order—#1 matters the most, #18 matters the least—for how each value matters to you, or rather, how much each value is a guiding principle in your life. It is important to prioritize these values according to the way things are for you, not based on how you believe you should prioritize the list, how others might prioritize it for themselves, or how they might prioritize it for you.

Now that you have taken a good inventory of your own values, tap into your values as a physical therapist or physical therapist assistant. The American Physical Therapy Association (APTA) details the Core Values[15] of the profession of physical therapy to help provide consistency in what society should expect from a physical therapy encounter. The following activity will highlight the values identified by the profession.

TABLE 1-1 (CONTINUED). ROKEACH VALUE SURVEY SAMPLE		
SAMPLE INSTRUMENTAL VALUES	**RANKING OF INSTRUMENTAL VALUES**	**WHAT IS THE MEANING OF THIS VALUE TO YOU? WHY DOES IT MATTER?**
Ambitious	1.	
Broad-minded	2.	
Capable	3.	
Clean	4.	
Courageous	5.	
Forgiving	6.	
Helpful	7.	
Honest	8.	
Imaginative	9.	
Independent	10.	
Intellectual	11.	
Logical	12.	
Loving	13.	
Loyal	14.	
Obedient	15.	
Polite	16.	
Responsible	17.	
Self-controlled	18.	
Reprinted with permission from Johnston, CS. The Rokeach Value Survey: Underlying structure and multidimensional scaling. *J Psychol.* 1995;129(5):583-597.		

Activity 1-6: Personal and Professional Core Values

Complete the *APTA Core Values Self-Assessment*[16] available at http://www.apta.org/Professionalism, or, if you are a physical therapist assistant, complete the *Values-Based Behaviors for the Physical Therapist Assistant (PTA) Self-Assessment.*[17] Reflect upon how your personal values that you identified in Activity 1-5 compare to the *APTA Core Values* or *Values-Based Behaviors for the Physical Therapist Assistant.* Identify any gaps, and reflect upon why those gaps may exist and what actions you can take to close them.

Lead With Heart

Authentic leaders lead with both their heads and their hearts. Leading with heart allows authentic leaders to develop dynamic, enduring relationships and loyalty. Some may view leaders who lead with their hearts as soft, or as being unable to make tough choices or hard decisions.[6] Yet, leading with heart is not soft at all and is quite difficult because it takes courage to act and behave in alignment to one's values and principles.

Leaders who lead in a way that is congruent or aligned with personal beliefs and values tap into their authenticity and credibility, both of which their followers ultimately desire.[9] In general terms, alignment occurs when parts are positioned appropriately in relation to each other. For example, if binocular lenses are out of alignment or become misaligned, then a viewer will see a blurred or double image. Leading yourself in a way that aligns the head and the heart in accordance with your values creates the clear image of your authentic self.

Another way to understand alignment, misalignment, and authenticity is to consider frameworks that dissect an individual's inner core, or sense of self, into parts. For example, one framework dissects an individual's core into 3 parts: a public or social self, a private self, and a deep inner self.[10] The *outward public* or *social self* is the part that an individual demonstrates openly with others in social situations. The *private self* is an aspect of an individual of which the individual is aware but does not show to others. The *deep inner self,* sometimes referred to as the *shadow side of self,* is the aspect of an individual that is not fully at the level of consciousness but still influences behaviors and decisions.

Two American psychologists, Joseph Luft and Harrington Ingham, created the Johari Window,[18] another framework used for understanding alignment and misalignment, in 1955. This framework is used to help people better understand their relationship with themselves as well as others by capturing information such as feelings, experiences, views, attitudes, skills, intentions, and motivation, within or about a person, in relation to others, from 4 perspectives:

1. What is known by the person about him- or herself and is also known by others—this is referred to as the *open area,* **open self,** *free area, free self,* or *arena.*

2. What is unknown by the person about him- or herself, but which others know—this is the *blind area,* **blind self,** or *blind spot.*

3. What the person knows about him- or herself that others do not know—this is the *hidden area,* **hidden self,** *avoided area, avoided self,* or *facade.*

4. What is unknown by the person about him- or herself and is also unknown by others – this is the *unknown area* or **unknown self.**

Activity 1-7: Johari Window

Access the Johari Window[18] survey at http://kevan.org/johari or search the internet for "Johari Window." You choose the words that you feel best describe you, and then you invite others to do the same for you. The most revealing aspect will most likely be your blind spots and will let you know where you are misaligned with your authentic self. Reflect on your results once you receive them.

Establish Enduring Relationships

Leaders are not effective on their own. Authentic leaders are relationship-focused and build a support team of people who value them for who they are and who can provide open and honest feedback during both good times and bad. These people may include family members, spouses or partners, friends, professional peers, coaches, and mentors. Regardless of the person, these individuals know the authentic leader well and are extremely valuable because they can provide the feedback that is needed for self-development and growth.

A-HA! – YOUR RELATIONSHIPS

Who is in your support team, and in what ways is each person valuable to your leadership development?

Support Team Member	Value of This Person to You

When do you usually access your support system (eg, when you have good news, when you need help, when you need emotional support)?

_____

_____

_____

From the activities that you have already completed in this chapter that encouraged you to obtain feedback from others, whom did you ask for the feedback, and why did you choose these people?

_____

_____

_____

What do you do regularly to support these valuable relationships that you have made?

_____

_____

_____

●————————————————

The support team that surrounds the authentic leader has also been found to be the primary factor in resilience,[19] another quality of the authentic and effective leader. *Resilience*, or hardiness, is the process of adapting well in the face of failure; hardship; trauma; significant stress resulting from family, relationship, or serious health problems; or workplace and financial challenges.[20] Resilience means bouncing back from difficult experiences, and it involves learning and developing specific behaviors, thoughts, and actions. Resilient people view a difficulty as a challenge, not as a paralyzing event. They look at their failures and mistakes as lessons from which they can learn and as opportunities for growth. They do not view failure as a negative reflection on their own abilities or self-worth. Resilient people are committed to their lives, their relationships, and their goals, and they have a compelling reason to get out of bed in the morning. Resilient people spend their time and energy focusing on situations and events in which they have control or influence. Because they put their efforts where they can have the most impact, they feel empowered and confident, as compared to individuals who spend time worrying about uncontrollable events, and who often feel lost, helpless, and powerless to act.

Developing resilience is a personal journey. An approach to building resilience that works for one person might not work for another because people do not react the same to traumatic or stressful life events. Additionally, through self-reflection, individuals can learn something about themselves and may find that they have grown in some respect as a result of their struggle with loss or failure.

Strategies to consider to build resilience[20] include:

- Making connections and keeping connected with close family members, friends, or others
- Accepting help and support from those who care about you and will listen to you
- Intentionally changing how you interpret and respond to crises or traumatic events

- Learning to accept change as an essential part of living
- Accepting circumstances that cannot be changed while focusing on circumstances that you can alter

A-HA! – RESILIENCE

Focusing on past experiences and sources of personal strength can help you learn resilience-building strategies that might work for you. By exploring answers to the following questions about yourself and your reactions to challenging life events, you may discover how you can respond effectively to difficult situations in your life.

What kinds of events have been most stressful for you, and why?

_____

_____

_____

_____

_____

How have those events typically affected you, and why?

_____

_____

_____

_____

_____

Have you been able to overcome obstacles? If so, how?

_____

_____

_____

_____

_____

Have you used your support team successfully through failures, or through traumatic or stressful experience? If so, how? If not, why not?

_____

_____

_____

_____

_____

Demonstrate Self-Discipline

Authentic leaders set high standards for themselves and accept full responsibility for outcomes. Committed to their personal values, authentic leaders have laser-focus and seemingly constant strength in the face of change and challenge. Two valuable assets for any authentic leader in the areas of self-discipline are the development of a personal mission statement and the development of a growth mindset.

An essential step in developing as a personal leader is to craft a personal mission statement. This will help you, as a personal leader, focus on what you want to be, and will encompass your core values that you have already identified earlier in this chapter. Covey describes a *personal mission statement* as "a personal constitution, the basis for making major, life-directing decisions, the basis for making daily decisions…"[10(p108)] Your personal mission statement can serve as your guide for self-discipline throughout your life. Sample personal mission statements are listed here to give you an idea of what other effective leaders have found important to them.

- Sample Mission Statement 1:
  - My mission is to be true to myself, to respect all others, and to always behave in a way that would make my mother proud.
- Sample Mission Statement 2:
  - My mission is to remember where I have been and where I will go through creating and maintaining positive relationships with family and friends.

Activity 1-8: Develop Your Personal Mission Statement

Developing a personal mission statement may sound like an easy task, but expect that completing this task will take time, honesty, and a great deal of introspection and reflection. One way to get started on your mission statement is to reflect back to the work you have already completed in this chapter to answer the following questions:

- What are you naturally good at? What strengths can you leverage? (Activities 1-1 and 1-2)
- What do you love about your life? Your work? Why? (A-Ha! – Discover Your Passion)
- Who has inspired you? Why? (Activity 1-4)
- What are your values? (Activity 1-5)
- When are you at your best? Your worst? Are you in alignment with your true self? (Activity 1-7)

Now summarize what you know about your authentic self to write your mission statement.

Another way to get started on your mission statement is to access one of the many internet sources dedicated to this task. One well-constructed guide is the mission statement builder available at http://msb.franklincovey.com that systematically walks you through the whole process.

A second attribute of the authentic leader in the areas of self-discipline is the development of a growth mindset. Mindset affects attitude, expectations, and behavior. Individuals who choose to be effective personal leaders have mindsets or beliefs about themselves and their most basic qualities, and adopt a view for themselves that deeply affects the way they lead their lives.[21] People in a *fixed* mindset believe their basic qualities, such as their intelligence or talent, are fixed traits, and believe that talent, not effort, creates success.[21] Leaders with a fixed mindset spend energy and time trying to prove their value to themselves and others, and if they fail, they see themselves as the failure.

Alternatively, people in a *growth* mindset believe that their most basic abilities can be developed through dedication, hard work, and intentional practice, and ultimately, this mindset fosters continuous learning and resilience. People—such as Mozart, Darwin, or Michael Jordan—identified with a growth mindset understood that it took years of passionate practice, attempts, failure, and learning to accomplish great things.[21] It takes self-discipline. Leaders with a growth mindset deliberately

TABLE 1-2. CHARACTERISTICS: PEOPLE WITH FIXED VERSUS GROWTH MINDSETS	
FIXED MINDSET	**GROWTH MINDSET**
Intelligence is static or fixed	Intelligence can be developed
Leads to desire to look smart and therefore has a tendency to:	Leads to desire to learn and therefore has a tendency to:
• Avoid challenges • Give up easily due to obstacles • See effort as fruitless • Ignore useful feedback • Be threatened by others' success	• Embrace challenges • Persist despite obstacles • See effort as path to mastery • Learn from peer feedback • Be inspired by others' success
Adapted from Dweck C. *Mindset: The New Psychology of Success.* New York, NY: Ballantine Books; 2008 and Waghorn T. Are You Trapped In A Fixed Mindset? Fix It! *Forbes.* https://www.forbes.com/2009/04/20/mindset-psychology-succcess-leadership-careers-dweck.html#c4eb0b211ada. Published June 19, 2013. Accessed September 25, 2018.	

invest time, energy, and practice to become more effective as leaders. A few key elements differentiating individuals with a growth mindset as compared to a fixed mindset are highlighted in Table 1-2.[21]

Similar to a growth mindset, an abundance mindset describes the mindset of a person who views situations from a win-win perspective and who believes enough resources and opportunities exist to share successes and recognition with others.[10] This mindset allows individuals to be excited by possibilities rather than limitations, and allows individuals to fail. According to Covey, the abundance mentality arises from within individuals who have a high self-worth and feel secure. In contrast, individuals with a scarcity mindset view situations from a win-lose perspective. In other words, only so many resources are available, and if others win, or gain access to these finite resources, then they lose.

Leaders' mindsets help determine how they think about and interpret situations, guide their emotional reactions, and influence decisions they make or actions they take. Essentially, leaders' mindsets set the tone for their ability to be self-disciplined and authentic.

Activity 1-9: Mindset Self-Assessment

Go to https://www.mindsetworks.com/assess and take the self-assessment[22] designed from the book *Mindset*, by Carol Dweck.[21] Once finished, determine how you could shift yourself from a fixed mindset to a growth mindset, or to a greater growth mindset than you already have, by doing the following:

- Think about an area in which you once struggled, but now you are proficient. How did you make the change? How can you apply this aptitude to other situations?
- List at least 3 situations in which you can choose to approach situations differently. Consider the following examples to get you started:
  - **When you approach a challenge.** The fixed mindset might say, "Am I confident I can do this? Maybe I don't have enough talent." Instead, the growth mindset answers, "I'm not completely confident I can do it now, but I know I can learn, and I'm willing to try."
  - **When you hit a setback.** The fixed mindset might say, "This would be easy if I just had the talent." Instead, the growth mindset says, "That was tough! But basketball wasn't easy for Michael Jordan, and inventing wasn't easy for Thomas Edison. They both had passion, they worked hard, and they put forth the effort."[23]

Bottom Line!

Ultimately, you cannot be authentic if you try to imitate someone else. Certainly, you can learn from others' experiences, but there is no way you can be truly effective as a leader if you try to be like them. People will trust you only if you are genuine and authentic, and not a replica of someone else. It takes work and commitment to become an authentic leader.

Case Study

Janet R. Bezner, PT, DPT, PhD, FAPTA

I was trained as a facilitator for Covey's *The 7 Habits of Highly Effective People* about 20 years ago, and in that process, we engaged in tremendous self-reflection about what was truly important to us (values) and how values differ from principles. The important point is that values should align with principles, and when they don't, values don't function very effectively to guide our personal decision-making.

If an individual doesn't know what's important to her, it's very difficult to make good decisions and live with integrity. My core values guide all of my decision-making—how I spend my time, the activities I chose to engage in and the ones I don't, how I build relationships, with whom I build relationships, etc. All of these issues are a part of leading oneself and leading others. People respect and follow others who stand for something and can articulate a vision—core values are prerequisites for developing passion and interest and achieving stretch goals.

I am a very direct person, and I often play the role of verbalizing what others are thinking but might not think should be said. Similarly, I have moral courage to stick up for what I think is right, even when it alienates me from others I care about. I can see the big picture and understand the value of something to a system or group, which can help people get unstuck when the personal ramifications of the issue become a barrier to solving problems. I have a high energy level and am highly productive, which I rely on to contribute in the many ways I desire to contribute.

My personal mission is to make everything I do or engage in better than I found it. Passion is hugely important for leadership because it helps get others excited about a vision, it supports an individual to take risks, it stretches the status quo to discover and develop new ways of doing things (to be innovative), and it fuels the ability to go in a different direction from the mainstream. Related to the profession, I am passionate about defining, expanding, and enhancing the value that physical therapy brings to society and that physical therapists bring to health care and to individuals. Within this larger vision, I specifically am very passionate about the role of physical therapists in increasing the physical activity of members of society.

This case study represents the story of an authentic leader. Now think again about your story that you started at the beginning of the chapter, and see what you can do to describe your authentic self.

Chapter Key Words

Leadership, Authenticity, Purpose, Passion, Storytelling, Principles, Values, Alignment, Resilience, Mission Statement, Mindset

References

1. Bonnstetter B, Suiter J. *The Universal Language DISC Reference Manual.* Scottsdale, AZ: Target Training International, Ltd.; 2013.

2. The Myers & Briggs Foundation. *Myers-Briggs Type Indicator.* https://www.myersbriggs.org/my-mbti-personality-type/mbti-basics/the-16-mbti-types.htm?bhcp=1. Accessed October 21, 2018.

3. DISC Assessment. *Insights2Improvement.* http://www.insights2improvement.com/About-Insights-2-Improvements.html. Accessed October 21, 2018.

4. CliftonStrengths. *CliftonStrengths.* https://www.gallupstrengthscenter.com. Accessed October 21, 2018.

5. CliftonStrengths Theme Quick Reference Card. *CliftonStrengths for Students.* https://www.strengthsquest.com/192458/clifton-strengths-theme-quick-reference-card.aspx. Accessed October 21, 2018.

6. George B, Sims P. *True North: Discover Your Authentic Leadership.* 1st ed. San Francisco, CA: Jossey-Bass; 2007.

7. Northouse PG. *Introduction to Leadership: Concepts and Practice.* Thousand Oaks, CA: SAGE Publications; 2017.

8. Kouzes JM, Posner BZ. *The Leadership Challenge: How to Make Extraordinary Things Happen in Organizations.* 5th ed. San Francisco, CA: Jossey-Bass; 2012.

9. Kouzes JM, Posner BZ. *The Leadership Challenge: How to Make Extraordinary Things Happen in Organizations.* 6th ed. Somerset, NJ: John Wiley & Sons, Inc.; 2017.

10. Covey SR. *The 7 Habits of Highly Effective People: Restoring the Character Ethic.* First Fireside edition. New York, NY: Fireside Book; 1990.

11. Brown B. *The Gifts of Imperfection: Let Go of Who You Think You're Supposed to Be and Embrace Who You Are.* City Center, MN: Hazelden; 2010.

12. Bezner J. Testimonial excerpted from original chapter case study. October 2014.

13. Sinek S. *Start With Why: How Great Leaders Inspire Everyone to Take Action.* London, UK: Penguin Business; 2009.

14. Johnston CS. The Rokeach value survey: underlying structure and multidimensional scaling. *J Psychol.* 1995;129(5):583-597.

15. American Physical Therapy Association. *Professionalism in Physical Therapy: Core Values.* http://www.apta.org/Professionalism. Accessed March 21, 2020.

16. American Physical Therapy Association. *Professionalism in Physical Therapy: Core Values Self-Assessment.* http://www.apta.org/Professionalism. Accessed October 19, 2018.

17. American Physical Therapy Association. *Values Based Behaviors for Physical Therapist Assistants.* http://www.apta.org/ValuesBasedBehaviors. Accessed October 21, 2018.

18. Johari Window. https://kevan.org/johari. Accessed October 21, 2018.

19. Kobasa SC. Stressful life events, personality, and health: An inquiry into hardiness. *J Pers Soc Psychol.* 1979;37(1):1-11. doi:10.1037/0022-3514.37.1.1

20. American Psychological Association. *The Road to Resilience.* http://www.apa.org/helpcenter/road-resilience.aspx. Accessed September 25, 2018.

21. Dweck C. *Mindset: The New Psychology of Success.* New York, NY: Ballantine Books; 2008.

22. Mindset Works. *What's My Mindset? (For Age 12 to Adult).* https://www.mindsetworks.com/assess. Accessed March 21, 2020.

23. Waghorn T. *Are You Trapped In A Fixed Mindset? Fix It!* Forbes. https://www.forbes.com/2009/04/20/mindset-psychology-succcess-leadership-careers-dweck.html#c4eb0b211ada. Published June 19, 2013. Accessed September 25, 2018.

SUGGESTED READINGS

Clifton DO, Harter JK. *Investing in Strengths*. Princeton, NJ: The Gallup Organization; 2003. http://media.gallup.com/documents/whitepaper--investinginstrengths.pdf. Accessed July 30, 2018.

Covey SR. *The 7 Habits of Highly Effective People: Restoring the Character Ethic*. First Fireside edition. New York, NY: Fireside Book; 1990.

Dweck C. *Mindset: The New Psychology of Success*. New York, NY: Ballantine Books; 2008.

George B, Sims P. *True North: Discover Your Authentic Leadership*. 1st ed. San Francisco, CA: Jossey-Bass; 2007.

Discovering Your Influence and Capacity to Become an Effective Personal Leader

Jennifer Green-Wilson, PT, MBA, EdD

Stacey Zeigler, PT, DPT, MS

So the point is not to become a leader. The point is to become yourself, to use yourself completely—all your skills, gifts, and energies—to make your vision manifest. You must withhold nothing. You must, in sum, become the person you started out to be, and enjoy the process of becoming.[1(p106)]

— *Warren G. Bennis*, On Becoming a Leader

CHAPTER OBJECTIVES

- Define *personal leadership*.
- Discuss characteristics of ineffective leaders.
- Discuss characteristics of effective leaders.
- Define *influence*.
- Discuss the link between influence and leadership.

Green-Wilson J, Zeigler S, eds.
Learning to Lead in Physical Therapy (pp 23-37).
© 2020 Taylor & Francis Group.

Leadership Vignette

Jerre van den Bent, PT

Several years ago, I had a life-changing experience relating to leadership. I attended a conference for physical therapists in Tacoma, Washington, on autonomous practice and leadership. Physical therapists from across the profession shared their thoughts and experiences on what it takes to be an effective leader. Despite being in a formal leadership position as an owner, I still struggled with a few issues in my pediatric home-care business and decided that this conference would give me ideas for improving the way I led my team. At the time, I did not understand the fundamental difference between leadership and management. My takeaway from this conference was that leadership and management are not about personality, but rather the skills, strategy, and knowledge of the leader. Furthermore, leadership and management can both be learned. Immediately after the conference with to-do list in hand, I got to work. Within 3 or 4 months, I had read 9 or 10 of the leadership books that had been recommended during the conference. Today, I make major decisions for my business and my team based on what I learned from the people I met at this conference and from the information I have subsequently read.

Recently, I encountered another discovery about leadership after attending the LAMP-leadership program sponsored by HPA The Catalyst, where LAMP stood for Leadership; Administration; Management; and Professionalism, Policy, or Practice. From this new program, called "Lead Wherever You Are: Becoming a Personal Leader," I came away with new inspiration and a better understanding of what leadership means in terms of opportunity. This time, I passed along what I learned, including my reading assignments, to my team of directors. Now, I am more effective as a formal leader because I have spent time developing my own leadership skills, and I am more aware of why I am effective. I manage myself better, which includes developing my personal mission statement, and more carefully in aligning my interests. I realize the importance of developing influence as a leader, and am more confident with my ability to know how and when to interact with others to increase my influence. My personal leadership style is about personal selling. For example, when I ask my employees or some of my colleagues to do something, I make sure to explain my reason for asking (the "why") and how they benefit from the "ask."

Understanding how to influence others is a vital skill for any future leader to learn. Leading is influencing. Many of us are influential, whether we understand why we are or not; however, understanding why and how we influence is important, as it can help preserve long-lasting relationships and professional success.

PERSONAL LEADERSHIP

It is critical to clarify what leadership is, and what it is not, and to identify the specific skills and behaviors that will demonstrate effective leadership at all levels in clinical practice. The term *personal leadership* describes leadership of self as an individual—the act of leading from within or leading from the inside to the outside. Personal leadership means informal leadership—you do not need a formal role, title, or responsibility to lead. Personal leadership means you can lead from wherever you are—from all levels—and make an impact.

Personal leadership is different from positional or formal leadership. The first distinction is to view leadership as behavior, and not as a formal title, position, role, or responsibility. When personal leadership is viewed as behavior, then the second distinction is to acknowledge that the first person you lead is you! Leadership is not about how to lead or change *others*, but how to lead or change *yourself.* This distinction highlights the essential need for personal leaders to develop their own personal leadership style or personal competence in how they interact with others.

Ultimately, leadership is about relationships, and your style of leadership impacts and influences your relationship dynamics in many ways. This requires you to choose purposefully to act in specific ways to be, do, and think, so you can be the best version of yourself. Personal leadership development requires you to hold up your own mirror to develop greater self-awareness and a better understanding of your own core—your values, beliefs, and passions that fuel your ability to demonstrate effective leadership behaviors at all times. This chapter is intended to help you develop your personal leadership through examination of your leadership characteristics.

INFLUENCE

Leadership means social influence in which the relationships between leaders and their followers, such as their peers, are crucial. Viewing leadership as dynamic relationships between people who work together to achieve shared outcomes applies well to physical therapist practice. Throughout this book, these cooperative relationships between physical therapists as personal leaders and their followers (ie, patients/clients) and other stakeholders (ie, peers, physical therapist assistants, and other members of the health care team) will be emphasized. By focusing on and identifying the key elements of these interactive leader-follower relationships, it will become clear how you can learn to lead effectively at all levels of clinical practice. In addition, you will learn how to influence others—or rather, how to interact with people most successfully—to achieve common goals and common interests, such as patient/client outcomes and behavioral change.

A-HA! – WHAT KIND OF INFLUENCE ARE YOU?

How do you define *influence*?

_____

_____

_____

What kind of influence are you **on yourself** (ie, positive, negative, aren't sure, or it depends), and why?

_____

_____

_____

Do you tend to focus your energy on things that are within your control to change, or do you tend to worry about things outside of your control?

_____

_____

_____

Does your self-talk include mostly statements starting with "I can" and "I will," or do you find yourself saying "I have to," "I should," or "If only I could"?

_____

_____

_____

If you aren't sure, pay attention to how you think and act over the next several days by keeping a log of your thoughts, feelings, and behaviors. You might be surprised at what you find.

————●————————————

Your answers to the questions listed previously begin the process of understanding the impact that you have on yourself every day. Leadership is about influence. If you are not a positive influence on yourself, then you will not be able to positively influence others. Stephen Covey, in his book *The 7 Habits of Highly Effective People*, developed an excellent visual model portraying that the larger you can increase your circle of influence (focusing energy and effort on things that are under your control), the more effective you will become as a leader.[2] On the flip side, spending your time and energy on negative self-talk or on issues that you have no control over will reduce your effectiveness and your capacity to influence.

This chapter will focus on effective and ineffective characteristics of leaders. It starts with a basic understanding of the effective and ineffective influence you have on yourself, and the influence you have noticed that others have on you. Often, it is easier to start this process by identifying behaviors and characteristics of an ineffective influencer than to identify the characteristics of an effective one. For example, have you worked with someone who is always negative and seems to be in crisis mode all the time? What about someone who hovers over your every move, critiquing you along the way, in such a way that you start to second-guess yourself? If you have ever experienced ineffective influence firsthand, then these encounters may still linger deeply in your memory because of the ways in which this upset you or made it difficult for you to do your work. Usually, after you reflect on these negative experiences, you can then start to see the opposite behaviors, or behaviors of effective actions, that would have made these relationship interactions more productive, satisfying, and enjoyable, and may even have contributed to your becoming a better person.

Activity 2-1: Ineffective and Effective Influencers

List a few behaviors or characteristics you have noticed in those you believe to be ineffective and effective influencers. In the right column, reflect on how these characteristics impacted you or the group. Try to discern why these characteristics impacted you. You will come back to your responses several times in this chapter, so make your list as complete as you can.

Ineffective Influencer Observations	Impact on You or the Group, and Why
Effective Influencer Observations	**Impact on You or the Group, and Why**

Now think about a situation when you had the opportunity to influence yourself (that is pretty much every moment of every day). Was the impact effective, or what could you have changed to improve the outcome, and why?

Something influences all of our behaviors. Whether it is our own self-talk or mindset, our past experiences, our environment, or other people with whom we may or may not interact, influence is ever-present. As we transition to the discussion of characteristics of effective and ineffective leadership, you will see how the 2 are nearly interchangeable: leadership is influence, and influence is leadership. The challenge is to ensure that your personal development in influencing yourself effectively translates to leading yourself effectively as well.

Bottom Line!

Authentic leadership cannot be bestowed, chosen, or assigned. Leadership only comes from influence, and influence must be learned.[3]

CHARACTERISTICS OF INEFFECTIVE LEADERS

How many of the ineffective influencer characteristics that you listed in Activity 2-1 were displayed by someone in a formal positional leadership role? It is not uncommon for each of us to have experienced working with a leader who displays ineffective, or even destructive, leadership characteristics. Fortunately, if you take time to understand why these interactions were not successful, you can learn from these experiences.

In Chapter 1, you used the Johari Window[4] as a mechanism for discovering your personal blind spots. Similarly, Zenger and Folkman have identified common shortcomings, flaws, or blind spots of leaders, specifically, 10 "fatal flaws" including[5]:

1. Lacking energy and enthusiasm
2. Accepting and remaining comfortable with their own mediocre or average performance
3. Lacking clear vision and direction
4. Having poor judgment
5. Not collaborating or cooperating with others
6. Not walking the talk (ie, saying one thing and doing something else)
7. Resisting new ideas
8. Not learning from mistakes
9. Lacking interpersonal skills
10. Failing to develop others

There are different types of ineffective leaders, and all types are frustrating to follow.[6] The ineffective leader is a leader no one wants to follow.[6] Ineffective leaders are also typically perceived as not being trustworthy. They are often seen as operating with questionable integrity, failing to consult with others for input, communicating poorly (if at all), ignoring problems, and not making decisions or addressing conflict.

When a leader does not display passion, enthusiasm, or commitment toward the team's vision yet expects everyone else to be passionate and committed to achieve certain outcomes, most likely, team members and followers will become disillusioned and discouraged by the "do what I say, not what I do" approach. When a leader tends to be mostly negative, reactive, and always in crisis mode (even when the issues are not close to being at a crisis level), the team's morale will go down. Often, team members will become worn out by a leader's negative approach. Additionally, when people follow a chameleon-type leader, they may waste valuable time and energy trying to predict and anticipate their leader's next move because they never know how the leader will react.[6] If a leader wants to spark innovation and change but makes fun of someone who has tried something new and did not succeed, then this leader's reaction may squash any momentum needed to fuel future initiatives.

A-HA! – YOUR LEADERSHIP CHARACTERISTICS

Leaders need followers, and your first follower is you! Consider how you lead yourself, and whether the characteristics you display are effective for your personal leadership development, and then answer these questions.

Which of your personal characteristics seem effective for leading yourself well?

_____

_____

_____

Which are less effective or ineffective characteristics?

_____

_____

_____

Would you follow you as a leader? Why or why not?

_____

_____

_____

If you need help knowing what characteristics you display, ask someone who works with you quite often, then see how many of these characteristics match the ones you have identified in the table of effective and ineffective characteristics in Activity 2-1.

CHARACTERISTICS OF EFFECTIVE LEADERS

Work has been done in the study of leadership to help isolate the characteristics of effective leaders. The most established of these characteristics are described, including how effective leaders are[2,7]:

- Authentic
- Passionate
- Proactive
- Emotionally intelligent
- Relationship builders
- Trustworthy
- Credible
- Future-oriented

Authentic

You have already started to discover your authentic self from the activities in Chapter 1. This is important, since numerous authors have noted that effective leaders display character or integrity and authenticity.[1,2,8] Effective leaders know themselves deeply; understand their strengths, weaknesses, and blind spots; and can leverage their strengths, minimize their weaknesses, and offset their blind spots in different situations. These leaders appear to have a distinct voice or a way to display their unique abilities with confidence but without an ego or arrogance, of being who they are inside-out without having to apologize or to change only to please others, and of being emotionally intelligent or capable of managing their relationships extremely well.[1]

Passionate

Passion is a deep and strong feeling about something. It is an intense emotion—a captivating enthusiasm or desire—that shapes your purpose or mission. Your passion influences not only who you are, but also with whom you connect and what opportunities you pursue. Passion fuels everything—from motivation to action to achievement. You know you are passionate about something when you become twitchy, when you wake up every morning knowing exactly what you have to do or who you have to be.[9]

People want to follow a passionate leader. Passionate leaders take the biggest risks, step up to the plate, and move teams forward. Passionate leaders ignite an emotional connection between people that becomes powerful, so that people working together can relate to each other through authenticity and trust. This very dynamic—shared emotional connection—sparks innovation and fuels change. Shared passion motivates people, gives them the sense of belonging, and excites them about being a part of a team.

Proactive

S. Covey suggests that effective leaders display behaviors that are proactive, not reactive.[2] Leaders who are proactive take initiative and are intentional about how they focus their time and energy and how they respond in different situations.[2] Being proactive means that individuals learning to lead create, shape, or control a situation to prevent something from happening or to cause something to happen in a particular way. Conversely, being reactive means waiting to respond to situations or outcomes until after they have happened.

You can become proactive by focusing more on the areas in which you can exert some control or influence instead of focusing on areas in which you cannot impact.[2] For example, if you are a student, you can become more proactive if you focus on completing assignments (something in your control) rather than focusing too much time worrying about the US economy or worldwide poverty (things less in your immediate control). By focusing time and energy on specific items within your area of influence or control, you can practice letting go of situations or concerns over which you have no ability to influence.

Emotionally Intelligent

Individuals learning to lead effectively can leverage their intelligence quotient (IQ), and they can also develop and use their emotional quotient (EQ). Highly effective leaders have a high degree of emotional intelligence that focuses on how they handle themselves and their relationships.[10] Your EQ is the capacity to deal strategically and proficiently with all sorts of emotions—your own, and those of others. One model used to delineate emotional intelligence, which may be helpful for developing leadership as a physical therapist, distinguishes among 4 domains and 18 associated competencies for emotional intelligence (Table 2-1).[10] This seminal work has recently been adapted using the original 4 domains, but now with 12 competencies rather than 18. Table 2-1 displays the original competencies, but the newer model, along with other valuable resources relating to emotional intelligence, can be accessed at www.keystepmedia.com.

Self-awareness and self-management (sometimes referred to as *self-regulation*) are classified as the 2 domains comprising personal competence or the capacity to manage yourself. Social awareness and relationship management (sometimes referred to as *social skill*) are classified as the domains

TABLE 2-1. FOUR DOMAINS AND ASSOCIATED COMPETENCIES OF EMOTIONAL INTELLIGENCE	
DOMAIN	**ASSOCIATED COMPETENCIES**
Personal Competence: Capabilities that determine how you manage yourself	
#1 Self-Awareness	Emotional self-awareness Accurate self-assessment Self-confidence
#2: Self-Management	Emotional self-control Transparency Adaptability Achievement Initiative Optimism
Social Competence: Capabilities that determine how you manage your relationships	
#3: Social Awareness	Empathy Organizational awareness Service
#4: Relationship Management	Inspirational leadership Influence Developing others Change catalysts Conflict management Building bonds Teamwork and collaboration

Reprinted with permission from Goleman D., Boyatzis R., McKee A. *Primal Leadership: Learning to Lead With Emotional Intelligence.* Boston, MA: Harvard Business School Press; 2002:39.

needed for achieving social competence or the capacity to manage your diverse social relationships and networks. Learning to lead requires that you focus on developing your personal competence first, and this starts with developing your self-awareness. Self-awareness requires becoming aware of your own emotions, and then paying attention to how your emotions and your emotional responses impact others.

Activity 2-2: Assess Your Emotional Intelligence

Review the competencies in Table 2-1, and then answer the questions in Table 2-2[10] as a start to identifying your EQ level.

Relationship Builders

Building and nurturing relationships takes hard work, time, and energy. Nevertheless, leading successfully is extremely dependent upon a leader's capacity to build and sustain many diverse relationships. In addition, the quality of a leader's relationships will directly impact the capacity of a

TABLE 2-2. EMOTIONAL INTELLIGENCE QUESTIONS

PERSONAL COMPETENCE

Self-Awareness/Self-Management

I understand how my emotions impact my ability to make decisions because I can read my emotions well.	Yes	Somewhat	Not at All
I know my strengths and my limitations or blind spots.	Yes	Somewhat	Not at All

Self-Management/Self-Regulation

I am able to keep disruptive emotions and impulses under control.	Yes	Somewhat	Not at All
I am flexible in adapting to changing situations or overcoming obstacles.	Yes	Somewhat	Not at All

SOCIAL COMPETENCE

Social Awareness

I am able to sense others' emotions and understand their perspective.	Yes	Somewhat	Not at All
I can read the vibes, decision networks, and politics at the organizational level.	Yes	Somewhat	Not at All

Relationship Management

I guide and motivate with a compelling or inspiring vision.	Yes	Somewhat	Not at All
I cultivate and maintain a network of relationships.	Yes	Somewhat	Not at All

Adapted from Goleman D., Boyatzis R., McKee A. *Primal Leadership: Learning to Lead With Emotional Intelligence.* Boston, MA: Harvard Business School Press; 2002.

leader to cultivate engagement, empowerment, and subsequent outcomes. Therefore, to be effective, leaders must develop emotional intelligence in the realm of social intelligence to increase their relationship know-how. Social intelligence is displayed mostly unconsciously through empathy, intuition, and compassion, and a socially intelligent leader can learn to sense another person's feelings and then adjust how to interact appropriately based on this newly acquired interpretation.[10]

A-HA! – RELATIONSHIPS

What do you do to build new relationships with others. What are the behaviors you use, and why?

_____

_____

_____

What do you do to maintain or sustain relationships. What are the behaviors you use, and why?

_____

_____

_____

What do others do with you to impact your relationship with them—either positively or negatively? Why are some of these actions important to you?

_____

_____

_____

●────────────────

Trustworthy

Something happens to a relationship when there is a lack of trust or, even more so, when there is distrust. Consider a time when you may have distrusted someone, and then reflect upon how this impacted your relationship. Overall, distrust creates doubt and suspicion. Distrust develops in a leader-follower relationship when others suspect that the leader has a hidden agenda, or when people discover that the leader is acting selfishly or not acting in their collective best interests.[11] Alternatively, trust develops in relationships when motives are clear, honest, transparent, and based on mutual benefit. Trust is fundamental to building and sustaining relationships, and in the long run, *followership*, described as the capacity or willingness to follow a leader.[1,11] A framework identified by S.M.R. Covey, in his book *The SPEED of TRUST: The One Thing That Changes Everything*, suggests that relationship trust depends on specific behaviors—certain interactions between people—and these interactions can increase or decrease trust.[11] In this framework, behaviors such as demonstrating respect, creating transparency, clarifying expectations, practicing accountability, listening first, and keeping commitments were found to be common in high-trust leadership-follower relationships.[11] Leaders learning to lead can develop and use these behaviors to build more productive relationships.

S. Covey, in *The 7 Habits of Highly Effective People*, used the metaphor "emotional bank account" to provide a practical way to think about how you can link your specific behaviors with your ability to build trust and, ultimately, relationships.[2] This model may be helpful for physical therapists learning to lead. For example, physical therapists as clinician-leaders can assess the account balance or amount of trust accrued in any relationship at any moment in time. Certain behaviors are considered *deposit behaviors*, whereas others are considered *withdrawal behaviors*. Leaders make withdrawals from relationship (emotional bank) accounts when they behave in ways that destroy trust. Leaders make deposits into those accounts when they behave in ways that build trust.[2] For example, deposits that you can make to significantly increase the emotional account balance in a relationship include appreciating each person as a unique individual, paying attention to little things, displaying general courtesies, being kind, keeping commitments, showing personal integrity, and apologizing sincerely when/if a relationship withdrawal is made.[2] It is important to note that deposits and withdrawals are not always equal or opposite. This means that what constitutes a deposit to one person may not to another, and often, withdrawals are perceived to be larger and more significant than deposits.[2,11] In addition, sometimes the best way to build trust is to stop making withdrawals within a relationship.

A-HA! – TRUST SELF-AWARENESS

As a way to learn to lead and to become more self-aware, take a few minutes to answer the following questions:

Are you someone others trust, or distrust? Why?

_____

_____

_____

TABLE 2-3. SAMPLE SELF-ASSESSMENT STATEMENTS ON CREDIBILITY			
STATEMENT	YES	NO	SOMETIMES
I lie.			
I am disrespectful.			
I am selective in how I share information.			
I break commitments.			
I am quick to judge others.			
I keep my intentions hidden.			
I manipulate the situation to my benefit.			

What could you do differently to build greater trust in your relationships?

_____

_____

_____

Establishing credibility is an important part of trust development. Perhaps an action item for you is to improve your credibility with others as a way to improve their trust in you. Keep reading to learn how.

Credible

A leader's credibility is fundamental for effective leadership and for engaging in productive, connected, and dynamic relationships. Leaders who are credible do what they say they will do.[7] People need to believe in their leaders and must believe that their words can be trusted. When it comes to deciding whether a leader is believable, people first listen to their words, then they watch their actions.[7] Additionally, credible leaders follow through on promises, practice what they preach, and ensure that their actions are consistent with their words.[7] Fundamentally, credible leaders "walk the talk." As leaders learning to lead, you can develop and increase your credibility by expanding your integrity through honesty, and this will directly and positively impact the amount of trust in relationships.[11] You can also develop greater credibility when you are transparent in your motives and behaviors—what you do to inspire confidence and engagement, and to produce empowered results.[11] Finally, you can earn credibility by demonstrating a strong track record of performance.

Activity 2-3: Self-Assess Your Credibility

Answer the questions in Table 2-3.

Review your responses in Table 2-3. Did you respond honestly? Did you have to think about some of them before you answered? Would others complete the table about you the same way?

Recognizing how many "Yes" or "Sometimes" responses you have given indicates areas for growth as you progress with improving your credibility to build trust with others.

Future-Oriented

Now that you are starting to identify potential areas for improving your leadership characteristics, you are also starting to display another key characteristic of an effective leader: being future-oriented. Ideally and in general, effective leaders spend most of their time and energy envisioning—looking ahead, into the future. Being forward-looking is the second most-admired characteristic that people look for in leaders they choose to follow.[7] Leaders optimistically envision possibilities and opportunities—they can picture what could be—and then, they inspire everyone to work together toward that compelling vision and a common future. Effective leaders translate *visions*, ideas for the future, into reality and into specific steps for implementation. Additionally, effective leaders articulate their own passions in ways that fuel the imaginations in others about possibilities.[7]

Bottom Line!

Research informs that the characteristics of some of the most effective leaders include their authenticity, passion, proactivity, emotional intelligence, ability to build relationships, trustworthiness, credibility, and future-orientation. When deciding where to focus your energy for personal leadership development, these qualities are an excellent place to start.

A MODEL FOR EFFECTIVE LEADERSHIP

Another extensively researched model describing the characteristics of the most effective leaders comes from Kouzes and Posner in their book, *The Leadership Challenge: How to Make Extraordinary Things Happen in Organizations*.[7] These authors have found that the most effective leaders believe passionately they can make a difference, envision the future by creating an ideal and unique image of what the team or the organization can become, enlist others in these dreams, and get people to see exciting possibilities. Their model for exemplary leadership identifies the 5 practices exhibited by leaders, as well as 2 main commitments for each of the 5 practices. These are summarized in Table 2-4.[7]

Applying the model developed by Kouzes and Posner, you can assess how much you feel you exhibit the characteristics of effective or exemplary leaders. The *Leadership Practices Inventory* (LPI)[12] applies the principles of Kouzes and Posner's "The Five Practices of Exemplary Leadership®," and enables individuals to gain insight into how they see themselves as leaders, how others view them, and what actions they can take to improve their effectiveness as a personal leader. LPI self-assessments require a fee and can be found at: www.leadershipchallenge.com/professionals-section-lpi.aspx.

Bottom Line!

People are watching you, regardless of whether you know it or not. And you are having an impact on them, regardless of whether you intend to or not.... Leadership is about the actions you take.... You are accountable for the leadership you demonstrate. And because you are the most important leader to those closest to you (ie, your patients and your peers), you have to decide how good a leader you want to be.[7]

TABLE 2-4. FIVE PRACTICES AND 10 COMMITMENTS OF EXEMPLARY LEADERS

5 PRACTICES	10 COMMITMENTS
1. Model the Way Individuals learning to lead model the way by clarifying their values, finding their inner voice, and affirming shared ideals. These individuals set the example by aligning actions with shared values. Because leaders are always watched by others, leaders set the example by demonstrating or modeling behaviors they expect of others.[7]	1. Clarify your values by finding your voice and affirming shared ideals. 2. Set the example by aligning actions with shared values.
2. Inspire a Shared Vision Effective leaders allow for time and energy to envision the future, listen closely for shared ambitions, and recruit and enlist others to explore forward-looking opportunities together.[7]	3. Envision the future by imagining exciting and ennobling possibilities. 4. Enlist others in a common vision by appealing to shared aspirations.
3. Challenge the Process Effective leaders challenge the process and their teams by searching for opportunities to rock the boat or to change the status quo, and by looking for innovative ways to improve the organization or practice through risk-taking and experimentation.[7]	5. Search for opportunities; seize the initiative; look outward for innovative ways to improve. 6. Experiment and take risks through generating small wins and learning from experience.
4. Enable Others to Act Highly effective leaders have the ability to influence and engage others into action by building trust, facilitating relationships, and fostering collaboration.[1,7]	7. Foster collaboration by building trust and facilitating relationships. 8. Strengthen others by increasing self-determination and developing competence.
5. Encourage the Heart Effective leaders know the value to be gained by sincerely recognizing and honoring the contributions made by individuals, as well as acknowledging the small wins and positive steps achieved. By doing so, they help others feel valued and appreciated, and therefore help others stay actively engaged in moving forward collectively.[7]	9. Recognize contributions by showing appreciation for individual excellence. 10. Celebrate values and victories by creating a spirit of community.

Reprinted with permission from Kouzes J, Posner B. *The Leadership Challenge, How to Make Extraordinary Things Happen in Organizations.* 6th ed. San Francisco, CA: Jossey-Bass; 2017.

Case Study: Personal Leadership Development Action Plan

Many activities outlined in this chapter and throughout this book will help you realize your personal leadership capacity. Take a minute now to review and list the effective leadership characteristics that you possess and that you would like to strengthen to become a better leader. Go back to each activity and self-assessment in this chapter to create a concise summary here of your strengths and areas to improve. YOU are this chapter's case study! Now complete the action plan to establish a contract with yourself to begin your journey of effective personal leadership.

PERSONAL LEADERSHIP DEVELOPMENT CONTRACT

After discovering more about the importance of developing personal leadership skills, I am willing to make the following Personal Leadership Development Contract with myself:

I will do _____ [identify an action] because I want to _____ [identify why you want to build a strength or minimize a shortcoming]. This is important to me because _____ [identify your personal goal—what you want to develop or achieve by making this change].

I'll know that I have made progress when _____ [identify the ideal change in your behavior] and I will evaluate my progress in _____ [# of days or months].

If I have not made progress in this time, I will _____ [identify a follow-up action].

CHAPTER KEY WORDS

Leadership, Personal Leadership, Influence, Emotional Intelligence, Proactive, Trustworthy, Credibility, Self-Awareness, Self-Management, Social Awareness, Relationship Management, Vision, Followership

REFERENCES

1. Bennis WG. *On Becoming a Leader*. 20th anniversary ed., rev. and updated. New York, NY: Basic Books; 2009.

2. Covey SR. *The 7 Habits of Highly Effective People: Restoring the Character Ethic*. First Fireside edition. New York, NY: Fireside Book; 1990.

3. Maxwell JC. *The 21 Irrefutable Laws of Leadership: Follow Them and People Will Follow You*. Nashville, TN: Thomas Nelson Publishers; 1998.

4. Johari Window. https://kevan.org/johari. Accessed October 21, 2018.

5. Zenger J, Folkman J. Ten fatal flaws that derail leaders. *Harv Bus Rev*. 2009;87(6):18.

6. Maxwell JC. *The 360 Degree Leader: Developing Your Influence from Anywhere in the Organization*. Nashville, TN: Thomas Nelson, Inc.; 2005.

7. Kouzes JM, Posner BZ. *The Leadership Challenge: How to Make Extraordinary Things Happen in Organizations*. 6th ed. Somerset, NJ: John Wiley & Sons, Incorporated; 2017.

8. George B, Sims P. *True North: Discover Your Authentic Leadership*. 1st ed. San Francisco, CA: Jossey-Bass; 2007.

9. Sinek S. *Start With Why: How Great Leaders Inspire Everyone to Take Action*. London, UK: Penguin Business; 2009.

10. Goleman D. *Emotional Intelligence: Why It Can Matter More Than IQ*. London, UK: Bloomsbury; 1996.

11. Covey SMR. *The SPEED of TRUST: The One Thing That Changes Everything*. New York, NY: Simon & Schuster; 2006.

12. Leadership Practices Inventory. *The Leadership Challenge*. http://www.leadershipchallenge.com/professionals-section-lpi.aspx. Accessed October 21, 2018.

SUGGESTED READINGS

Covey SMR. *The SPEED of TRUST: The One Thing That Changes Everything*. New York, NY: Simon & Schuster; 2006, 2018.

Covey SR. *The 7 Habits of Highly Effective People: Restoring the Character Ethic*. First Fireside edition. New York, NY: Fireside Book; 1990.

Goleman D, Boyatzis R, McKee A. *Primal Leadership: Learning to Lead With Emotional Intelligence*. Boston, MA: Harvard Business School Press; 2002.

Kouzes JM, Posner BZ. *The Leadership Challenge: How to Make Extraordinary Things Happen in Organizations*. 6th ed. Somerset, NJ: John Wiley & Sons, Incorporated; 2017.

3

Developing Your Leadership Style

Jennifer Green-Wilson, PT, MBA, EdD

Leadership is not magnetic personality; that can just as well be a glib tongue. It is not "making friends and influencing people," that is flattery. Leadership is lifting a person's vision to higher sights, the raising of a person's performance to a higher standard, the building of a personality beyond its normal limitations.

— *Peter F. Drucker, writer, professor, and management consultant*

CHAPTER OBJECTIVES

- ‣ Define *leadership style.*
- ‣ Examine key characteristics of leadership styles.
- ‣ Define *followership.*
- ‣ Self-assess your leadership style.

Green-Wilson J, Zeigler S, eds.
Learning to Lead in Physical Therapy (pp 39-55).
© 2020 Taylor & Francis Group.

Leadership Vignette

Craig Moore, PT, MS, MBA

I remember stepping into a formal leadership role and recognizing that the leader before me was gregarious, sociable, and well-known. After a year of trying to be like him—emulating his style of leadership—I realized that I was never going to be like him. I knew my style of leadership was different, and that it was okay. Once I accepted this, I gravitated toward aspects of leadership that were natural and important to me. I discovered that I have a strong need to get things done as a leader, and I need to create a structure and vision for us to do our work. I realized I could still be the leader and not be expected to have all the solutions. Leveraging my belief that great leaders have a spiritual center that allows them to connect with people in authentic ways, I realized I was most comfortable and effective in a leadership role in which I could work one-on-one with people in a quiet, more introverted way rather than in groups or large social settings.

LEADERSHIP STYLES

Numerous theories of leadership have evolved over time. This has led to meaningful translation of leadership theories into leadership behaviors or styles. Think of your *leadership style* as a distinct way of expressing or conducting yourself; it is your unique pattern of behaviors. Converting leadership theories into leadership styles helps define a range of observable behaviors or approaches that individuals can use when they are interested in becoming more effective as leaders. Typically, the style reflects the individual's personal beliefs, values, mindsets, and preferences, as well as representing an organization's culture or norms that encourage some styles and discourage others. As you move on in this chapter and begin to explore classic, contemporary, and emotionally intelligent styles of leadership, it will be helpful to identify specific behaviors that you expect to observe when individuals demonstrate this particular style, and pay close attention to those styles that resonate with you.

CLASSIC LEADERSHIP STYLES

Authoritarian, democratic, and laissez-faire are considered to be classic styles exhibited by individuals in formal or informal leadership roles. In 1939, Kurt Lewin, with a group of researchers, investigated leadership styles, specifically in reference to decision making.[1] Interestingly, Lewin acknowledged that one of the most significant factors shaping an individual's style of leadership was how the person chose to make decisions. In this study, children were assigned to groups led by individuals who used an authoritarian, democratic, or laissez-fair leadership style. The leaders led the children in an arts and crafts project, while researchers observed the children's behavior in response to different leadership styles.

Activity 3-1: Behavioral Effect on Performance

Think of the last time you were part of a group activity where someone other than you took the lead. Write down a few things about the behaviors of that individual and how that person's behavior affected your performance.

_____

_____

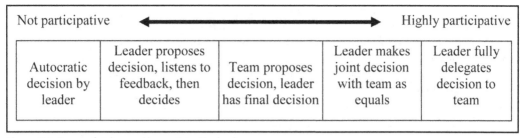

Figure 3-1. Range of styles used by participative leaders.

_____

_____

Now read on to determine if that person's leadership style was more authoritarian, democratic, or laissez-faire. At the end of this section, you will find out if your impressions match the results of the Lewin study.

Authoritarian (Autocratic) Leadership Style

An *authoritarian* is the type of person, such as a king or queen, who has undisputed positional influence or power, and who rules or commands with unlimited authority. Benito Mussolini, Adolf Hitler, and Vladimir Putin are examples of authoritarian leaders. Typically, authoritarian leaders do not involve others in the decision-making process. Rather, they make decisions independently, and, by doing so, are very efficient and perpetuate a well-defined division between the leader and the follower. Authoritarian leaders provide clear expectations for what, when, and how things need to be done. Also, once authoritarian leaders make a decision, they impose the decision on others and expect compliance. Interestingly, Lewin et al's experiments revealed that an authoritarian style works well when there is no need for input on a decision; specifically, in situations when input would not change a decision or outcome.[1] For example, in a crisis situation such as a fire in a building, a leader with an authoritarian style can be extremely effective at mobilizing a group toward safety. In this situation, there is no need for discussion or input, as the decision to evacuate as quickly as possible is clear.

Participative (Democratic) Leadership Style

Democratic leadership, also known as *participative leadership*, is a type of leadership style in which all members of the group participate in a shared decision-making process. Dwight D. Eisenhower is an example of a leader who predominantly used a participative leadership style. Even though participative leaders are recognized to involve others in decision making, they often maintain the final say. A leader with a participative style states the goal or the objective to be reached and then allows others to determine how the work will be done to achieve the intended goal. Figure 3-1 shows a range of styles participative leaders use depending on situational needs.

On the far right of the continuum, the participative leader delegates a decision to the team. In this scenario, the leader may bring the team together and ask team members to prepare a budget for the upcoming year. The team decides collectively how to determine what will be included in the budget, where to get information to support the budget, how to design the budget, how and who will provide input and also review the budget, and what deadlines must be established to finalize it. Alternatively, to the left of the continuum, the participative leader establishes a draft budget for the team to review. The leader encourages the team to ask questions, provide feedback, or possibly add new ideas or categories, and then the leader independently finalizes the budget using input gathered.

Because participative leaders believe people are more engaged and committed to action when they are involved in relevant decision making, these leaders consult others, share appropriate information and power, and facilitate collaborative decisions. Although others usually appreciate the participative leadership style of decision making, it can be inefficient and challenging in situations when there are many opinions and no clear directions on how to reach a decision that seems reasonable for all participants.

Laissez-Faire (Delegative) Leadership Style

A *laissez-faire* leadership style is characterized as non-authoritarian, or a hands-off approach. The French phrase *laissez-faire* broadly implies "let it be," "let them do as they will," or "leave it alone." Leaders with this style delegate to their followers and give little or no direction or guidance, even if asked. Leaders who use a laissez-faire style leave decision making to the group members, and generally do not get involved in the decision-making process themselves. Adam Smith, Thomas Jefferson, and Ronald Reagan are examples of laissez-faire leaders. Because a laissez-faire style allows team members to make their own decisions, it works best and is most effective when people are capable, motivated, and qualified to make these decisions, and when there is no need to collaborate or coordinate sharing resources across groups or people. However, if team members are missing critical information, knowledge, or skills, then this leadership and decision-making style may create havoc within and among teams through widespread indecision and confusion.

Activity 3-2: Results of Activity 3-1

Which of the 3 classic leadership styles matched best with the behaviors of your group work leader from Activity 3-1?

_____

_____

_____

Was the style effective for what you were doing?

_____

_____

_____

Did you feel that you performed your best with that style of leadership?

_____

_____

_____

The 1939 Lewin study found that democratic (participative) leadership appeared to be the most effective style, whereas authoritarian leadership and its subsequent style of decision making caused the highest level of discontent.[1] Children assigned to the laissez-faire leader were the least productive of all 3 groups, made more demands on the leader, showed little cooperation, and were unable to work independently.

How does your experience compare to this study's findings?

_____

_____

_____

The Lewin study focused on only one type of situation, children making crafts, but can you see how the findings may change under a different situation or task? Why or why not?

_____

_____

_____

Bottom Line!

All 3 classic leadership styles can be effective, and a single skilled leader may use all 3 styles within any given day based on the situation. The 3 classic leadership styles form the foundation of most styles used today, although they do not necessarily encompass every philosophy on how each situation requiring leadership should be handled.

CONTEMPORARY LEADERSHIP STYLES

What has been most consistent in the literature in recent times is the concept that leadership is about the behaviors that individuals exhibit and how adept individuals alter behaviors to meet situational demands. Both personal (informal) and formal leadership require an armament of styles greater than the 3 classics. This style armamentaria has become much broader and more defined, as you will now see with the exploration of the charismatic, quiet, transactional, situational, servant, and transformational leadership styles.

Charismatic (Extroverted) Leadership Style

An individual with a *charismatic leadership style* is described as someone who is charming, has a notable presence, and has a compelling appeal to others. Dr. Martin Luther King, Jr., a pioneer in the civil rights movement in the United States, is an example of a charismatic leader. King was renowned for his inspirational speeches, including the "I Have a Dream" speech he gave during the march on Washington, D.C., in 1963. His speech spurred people of all races to push for federal civil rights legislation. Charismatic leaders are proficient at connecting with people and can adapt their interpersonal styles and their charm to match different situations. They are approachable, likeable, captivating, and usually extroverted and sociable. An *extrovert* is typically characterized as outgoing or an overtly expressive person. Extroverts are usually most concerned with the physical and social environments rather than with the self.

Charismatic leaders are skillful at working a room by scanning their environments to read the moods, likes, and concerns of individuals as well as groups. Often, people are drawn to this alluring leadership style. People follow leaders whom they admire, and these leaders are successful at connecting and demonstrating confidence in their followers. Charismatic leaders are persuasive. They make valuable use of body language (nonverbal communication), verbal communication, and listening skills, and often use storytelling effectively. The values of the charismatic leader are highly significant, and as long as they are well-intentioned towards others, these leaders can elevate and transform an entire team or organization.

Activity 3-3: Are You Charismatic?

Do you display the charismatic style behaviors (eg, approachable, likeable, captivating, extroverted, persuasive, and sociable)? _____

If you aren't sure, ask someone who knows you.

If you want to increase your charisma, watch charismatic people in action, and take good notes! Study videos of charismatic leaders, their speeches, and the ways they interact with others, such as:

- Martin Luther King's "I Have a Dream" speech, available at www.youtube.com/watch?v=mAtOV_cp2b8
- Matthew McConaughey's "We Are Marshall—We Cannot Lose" speech, from the movie *We Are Marshall*, available at: www.youtube.com/watch?v=IEL8PYu4RR4

Quiet (Introverted) Leadership Style

Many people lead and influence others quietly, from behind the scenes.[2-4] Quiet or introverted leaders are the opposite of the charismatic or extroverted leaders. *Introverts* are typically characterized by needing time to recharge their batteries once having engaged in activities with other people. Introverts expend energy working with others, while extroverts gain energy. When associated with the term *quiet*, introvert does not mean speaking less, but rather, it refers to using quiet action to lead others. Quiet leaders lead by example; they do not tell people what to do, nor do they give elaborate speeches. Rather, they do what needs to be done, and encourage their followers to do the same. Quiet or introverted leaders focus on tasks, pay attention to core values, influence people through kindness and logical arguments, are selfless, display emotional control, and are bluntly realistic about the complexities of their own challenges and other problems they face.[2-4] Rosa Parks and Abraham Lincoln are examples of quiet leaders.

Activity 3-4: Quiet Versus Charismatic

Do you think the quiet or charismatic style sounds more like your natural style? The following activity may help. Read the descriptions listed in Group A and in Group B, then ask yourself which group of descriptions seems more comfortable, natural, and effortless for you:

- Group A:
  - I am seen as outgoing and a people person.
  - I feel comfortable in groups and enjoy working in them.
  - I have a wide range of friends; I know a lot of people.
  - I sometimes jump into an activity too quickly and do not allow enough time to think about it first.
- Group B:
  - I am seen as reflective and reserved.
  - I feel comfortable being alone; I enjoy doing things by myself.
  - I prefer to know just a few people well.
  - I sometimes devote too much time reflecting and do not move into action quickly enough.

If the descriptions from Group A speak to you the best, then you seem to be extroverted (a typical charismatic quality). On the other hand, if the descriptions from Group B speak to you, then you seem to be introverted (more of a typical quiet leadership style quality).

Transactional Leadership Style

The style of the transactional leader mirrors a style commonly used by managers, or formal leaders, who create clear structures to make performance expectations and rewards transparent, and then implement formal systems to isolate poor performance or the need for disciplinary action. Leaders who use a transactional style operate mainly on the following assumptions: people are motivated by reward and punishment, social systems work best when there is a clear chain of command for communication and decision making, people surrender authority to their leader or manager, and the team members' primary purpose is to follow instructions and act in a manner that helps achieve the goals for the group. Thus, the transactional leader frequently adopts more of a telling or directing style in working with others. It's a very black-and-white style of operating.

Transactional leaders rely on contingency, meaning that they reward or punish team members based on performance. Often, the transactional leader uses *management by exception*, operating on the principle that if someone meets performance expectations, then that person does not need attention from the leader. If performance exceeds expectations, then the leader provides praise and reward for exceptional work. However, if performance falls below expectations, then the leader applies corrective actions or some other form of consequence.

Activity 3-5: Transactional Leadership

Do you relate to the transactional style of leadership? Why or why not?

_____

_____

_____

Brainstorm how the transactional style may be effective or ineffective in different situations.

_____

_____

_____

Situational Leadership Style

Thus far, you have discovered that effective leaders can use different styles depending on situational needs. Individuals who exhibit *situational leadership styles* are adept at recognizing and using different styles at different times, and move from one style to the next with ease. The best style depends on the situation. Forces that influence a situational leader's behavior or style at a particular moment in time include:

- Dynamics of a specific situation
- Needs and developmental level (readiness) of the follower
- Adaptability of the leader

Effective situational leaders are successful when they adapt their leadership style to match the maturity or readiness of the individual or group they are attempting to lead or influence. A model for situational leadership, as portrayed in Figure 3-2,[5] identifies situations in which a particular leadership style aligns the best with the follower's need or level of readiness.[5] As you can see, no single leadership style is the best or considered optimal for all leaders to use all the time; the best style depends on the situation.

Looking at the model in Figure 3-2, the amount of Task Behavior (x-axis) relative to Relationship Behavior (y-axis) that a leader should provide to a follower (individual or group) becomes apparent after the leader determines the follower's maturity level or level of readiness to take on a particular task. *Task behavior* is described as the extent to which the leader engages in spelling out duties and responsibilities of an individual or group. Specific task-like behaviors include telling people what to do, how to do it, when to do it, where to do it, and who is to do it. *Relationship behavior* is described as the extent to which the individual who is leading engages in 2-way (or multi-way) communication while working with others. These relationship-like behaviors include listening, encouraging, facilitating, providing clarification, and giving support as needed. Furthermore, in this model, maturity reflects the follower's capacity to set high but attainable goals, the willingness and ability to take responsibility for a task, and the relevant education and/or experience needed by an individual or a group to perform the task. Essentially, the correct leadership style will depend on the person or group being led.

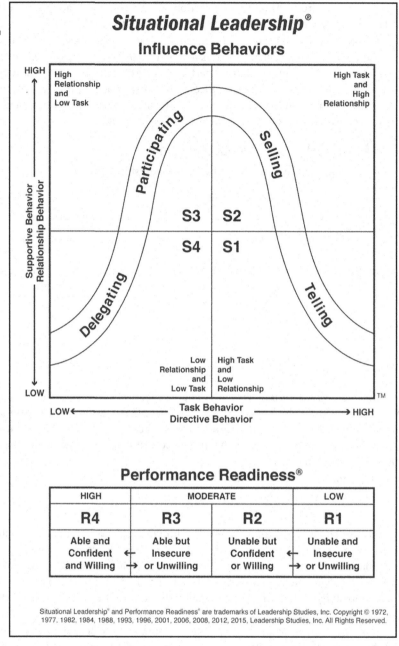

Figure 3-2. Framework for understanding situational leadership. (Reprinted with permission from Hersey P. *The Situational Leader.* San Diego, CA: The Center for Leadership Studies; 1984. 61, 67.)

In Figure 3-2, you will see 4 levels of follower maturity listed from M1 through M4 (or, sometimes referred to as R1 through R4) to indicate follower readiness. At level M1/R1, the follower is novice yet enthusiastic. These followers need help, guidance, and direction from their leader because they are not ready to take on full responsibility for the task. In this situation, the leader uses a *telling* leadership style (S1), characterized by one-way communication, in which the leader defines the roles of the individual or group and provides clear direction as to the what, how, why, when, and where to complete the task. At level M2/R2, the followers are still unable and unwilling to assume full responsibility because they lack specific skills or knowledge required to complete this particular task. At this level, the leader uses a *selling* style (S2) to still provide direction, and uses 2-way communication to provide support. This approach allows the individual or group to buy into the process a bit more. At the M3/R3 level, followers are experienced and capable to do the task, but still lack confidence or willingness to take on full responsibility. At this level, the leader uses a "participative" style of leadership (S3) characterized by less task-focused behavior, more relationship-focused behavior, and an approach to decision making that is more collaborative regarding how the task will be accomplished. At level M4/R4, followers are experienced at completing the task, comfortable with their ability to do it well, and willing to take on full responsibility for the task itself. The leader uses a "delegating" style at this level (S4), where the decision-making authority and any associated responsibility for a particular assignment are shared or transferred from the person leading to a specific member or members on the team. In this situation, the leader is still involved in decision making and monitors progress from time to time, but the process and responsibility have more or less been handed over to the individual or group.

Effective leaders need to remain flexible and be willing to adapt their own leadership style according to the situation. The situational leadership model provides a pragmatic tool to help new leaders learning to lead begin to know when and how to adapt their style when working with others. For example, if someone new joins your group, and your team has a deadline approaching, most likely as the team leader, you would adopt a telling or authoritarian style (S1) to align with the need for a high-task/low-relationship approach in this situation. However, if there is no imminent deadline and the two of you have worked on a few projects together, you might use more of a participative leadership style instead because you have had experience working together in the past, you are familiar with each other's strengths and areas of expertise, and you have more time to develop a collaborative relationship.

Activity 3-6: Situational Leadership Experience

Write an example of a time when you have demonstrated the situational leadership style.

_____

_____

_____

You probably did not even realize that you adapted and changed your style based on the need. Or perhaps in looking back, there was a circumstance that you can think of when you should have, but didn't, adapt.

Servant Leadership Style

Servant leaders focus primarily on the needs of others rather than how others can serve or follow the leader.[6] Servant leaders assume responsibility for followers, put followers' needs before their own needs, and connect with followers in a variety of ways so that, ultimately, the group can achieve, flourish, and improve. The style of the servant leader is characterized by empathy, listening, forethought, imagination, stewardship, the ethical use of power and empowerment, and community-building. Servant leaders cultivate relationships based on trust, and this foundation of trust encourages collaborative work and service.

Sir Ernest Shackleton was an explorer who led 3 British expeditions to the Antarctic and is an example of a servant leader. The Shackleton expedition (1914 to 1916) began with the mission of exploration, but turned into a mission of survival due to repeated disaster. After his ship froze in the Antarctic, Shackleton brought his entire 27-member crew home alive in open boats across the wintry Antarctic seas 2 years and 800 miles later. It was Shackleton's leadership style and his unwavering sense of responsibility toward his men that kept his fleet together in such extreme circumstances.

Activity 3-7: Are You a Servant Leader?

Does the servant leadership style resonate with you?

Compare and contrast the behaviors of the servant leader with the American Physical Therapy Association's *Core Values of Professionalism*[7] (accountability, altruism, caring/compassion, excellence, integrity, professional duty, and social responsibility) from Activity 1-6 in Chapter 1.

_____

_____

_____

Think of your relationships with patients/clients and your role as leader for that person. How does servant leadership apply to patient care and physical therapist practice?

_____

_____

_____

Transformational Leadership Style

Transformational leadership happens when both leaders and followers interact in ways that move each other to higher levels of conviction, engagement, and motivation.[8] The National Center for Healthcare Leadership defines *transformation* as "visioning, energizing, stimulating a change process that unites communities, patients/clients, and professionals around new models of healthcare and wellness."[9] In these dynamic leader-follower relationships, both the leader and the followers find meaning and purpose in their work, and both grow and develop from their relationship.

The style of the transformational leader has been described as uplifting, passionate, and energizing. These leaders demonstrate care for others; display a duty to help others succeed; and earn trust, respect, and admiration from their followers in such a way that their followers make a conscious choice to follow them as the leader—and that choice makes for a significant, dynamic bond.[8] Transformational leaders are proficient at leveraging the strength of their vision and personality to inspire followers to change expectations, perceptions, and motivations to work toward common goals.

Transformational leaders exude energy and passion in such a way that their followers become engaged and re-engaged to keep an ongoing, high level of commitment to the vision. These leaders are often charismatic, extroverted, and visible, remaining upfront and present during most of the group's activities. Their unwavering and energetic commitment motivates others, particularly through tough and challenging times when others may start to doubt whether the vision can be achieved.

Walt Disney is an example of a transformational leader. Walt Disney was a charismatic innovator who had a vision that he made into a grand reality. He influenced and inspired many people throughout his lifetime His entertainment empire has developed into a multi-billion dollar television, motion picture, vacation destination, and media corporation. Among other assets, The Walt Disney Company owns vacation resorts, theme parks, water parks, hotels, motion picture studios, record labels, cable television networks, and a television network. In 2017, revenues at The Walt Disney Company totaled more than $55 billion dollars.[10]

Activity 3-8: The Transformational Leader in You

Review the Kouzes and Posner "Five Practices and 10 Competencies of Exemplary Leadership" (see Table 2-4) from Chapter 2.[11] This is an example of a model for transformational leadership. Now review your self-assessment of the 5 practices (see Table 2-5). If you did not do this self-assessment previously, take the time to do it now.

Write 3 things you could do right now to improve your skills for becoming a leader using a transformational leadership style.

_____

_____

_____

Bottom Line!

"Imagine contemporary leadership styles as an array of golf clubs in a golfer's bag. Over the course of the game, the golfer selects different clubs to use based on the situation or the demands of the pending shot. By selecting the right tool at the right time, the golfer adapts swiftly and effectively to each unique situation. Similarly, effective leaders learn to adapt their style to match the needs and demands of each new situation in an efficient manner."[13]
- Daniel Goleman, Author, "Leadership That Gets Results," *Harvard Business Review*

Emotionally Intelligent Leadership Styles

In Chapter 2, the concept of emotional intelligence (EQ) was introduced as the capacity to deal strategically with your own emotions and those of others. Highly effective leaders have a high degree of EQ. Goleman further identified his work with EQ by distinguishing capabilities of EQ that drive 6 styles of leadership; these emotionally intelligent leadership styles include coercive, visioning, affiliative, democratic, pacesetting, and coaching. In Table 3-1, a summary of the 6 leadership styles is provided, as well as the specific EQ competencies at the core of each style.

According to Goleman, styles of leadership affect the climate of a team or organization. The term *climate* is used to describe elements that are important among team members, including how much flexibility team members have to solve problems, how committed they feel to the shared goals, how much responsibility they feel to the team or organization, and the level of standards or performance to which they need to adhere.

The individual who uses a coercive leadership style controls by fear (eg, "do it my way or else!"). This person takes charge and does not welcome opinions that are different or contrary. This style can have a detrimental impact on climate, especially if the intensity and longevity of this coercive approach persist. The individual who uses a *visioning* leadership style has a persuasive ability to convey shared goals and to gain an enthusiastic commitment to a common vision. The individual who uses an *affiliative* leadership style is highly effective at establishing dynamic relationships and gives frequent, positive feedback to keep everyone engaged in achieving individual and collective goals. Followers tend to appreciate working alongside individuals who use this leadership style and are likely to remain loyal to the team, share information openly with others, and have high trust within their relationships. The individual who uses a *democratic* leadership style focuses on decision making through consensus. Consensus helps foster trust and an intense commitment to goals, strategies, and tactics. The individual who uses a pacesetter leadership style sets extremely high performance standards for every person on the team. This *pacesetter* leader is usually highly motivated, with strong technical skills, and continually pushes everyone to be faster, better, and more thorough. Unfortunately, this approach can unintentionally undermine the efforts and morale of team members, especially when the pacesetting is perceived as unrelenting and overwhelming.[13] The individual who uses a *coaching* leadership style is focused on developing people through cultivating new skills, and this style works best when followers are receptive to personal growth.

TABLE 3-1. EMOTIONALLY INTELLIGENT LEADERSHIP STYLES

LEADERSHIP STYLE	LEADER'S APPROACH; STYLE	STYLE IN A PHRASE	UNDERLYING EMOTIONAL INTELLIGENCE COMPETENCY	WHEN THE STYLE WORKS BEST
Coercive	Demands immediate compliance	"Do what I tell you."	Drive to achieve Initiative Self-control	In a crisis situation, to kick-start a turnaround, or to deal with a problem team member
Visioning	Mobilizes people toward vision	"Come with me."	Self-confidence Empathy Change catalyst	When change requires new vision or when clear direction is needed
Pacesetting	Sets high standards for performance	"Do as I do now."	Conscientious Drive to achieve Initiative	To get quick results from highly motivated and competent team
Coaching	Develops people for the future	"Try this."	Developing others Empathy Self-awareness	To help team members improve performance or develop long-term strengths
Affiliative	Creates harmony and builds emotional bonds and connections	"People come first."	Empathy Building relationships Communication	To heal rifts in a team or to motivate people during stressful circumstances
Democratic	Forges consensus through participation	"What do you think?"	Collaboration Team leadership Communication	To build buy-in, consensus To get input from valuable team members

Reprinted with permission from Goleman, D. Leadership That Gets Results. *Harv Bus Rev*, March-April 2000:78-90.

Pacesetting and coercive leadership styles leverage the EQ competencies of drive to achieve and initiate, whereas democratic and affiliative leadership styles leverage the EQ competency of communication. Note that affiliative, visioning, and coaching leadership styles leverage the EQ competency of empathy, and a democratic leadership style leverages the EQ competencies of collaboration and team leadership. Goleman suggests that individuals learning to lead can master 4 or more of these styles, especially visioning, democratic, affiliative, and coaching styles, with intentional practice. By doing so, they can foster a more effective work climate or environment to yield higher levels of performance.[13]

Activity 3-9: Your Emotionally Intelligent Leadership Style

To help you determine which of the emotionally intelligent leadership styles you are good at, and which you might want or need to develop further, take the quiz[14] at http://www.skillsyouneed.com/ls/index.php/325444.

> ## Bottom Line!
>
> Leaders who achieve strong performance do not use one leadership style only; rather, the most effective leaders adapt their styles to different situations and can demonstrate many distinct leadership styles—sometimes all in the same day! Whether leaders can do this effectively or not is the challenge.

When the Best Style of Leadership Is Followership

In Chapter 2, you were introduced to the concept of followership, or being an effective follower. Most people spend more time following than leading, and leadership cannot exist without followership. Leaders can gain insight into how to become more effective by understanding how and why people relate to certain styles of leaders, and why people choose to follow someone—or not. A follower pursues a course of action in common with a leader to achieve a common goal.[15] Effective followers are described as individuals who are independent, critical thinkers with highly developed integrity and competency; who display great commitment; and who function well in a change-oriented team environment.[16] Effective followers recognize their leader's authority and the limitations that authority imposes on their own actions, consider issues based on their merits, make their own decisions, embrace their own values, speak their minds, and hold themselves accountable for the consequences for their actions.[16]

A-HA! – FOLLOWING

Answer these questions to start to uncover some reasons when the best style of leadership may be following.

Why do people follow leaders?

_____

_____

_____

When do you decide to follow rather than to lead?

_____

_____

_____

What does it take to be an effective follower?

_____

_____

_____

Figure 3-3. A Framework for Followership.[15]

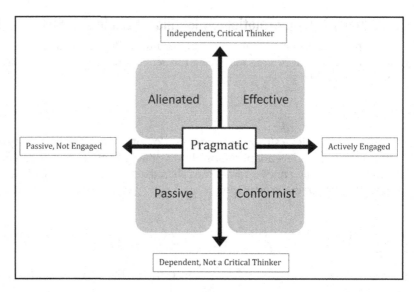

Two helpful dimensions in defining levels of followership include critical thinking and level of engagement.[15] Using these dimensions, effective followers are described as independent critical thinkers who are actively engaged and who generate positive energy for the team. They are not passive, do not produce negative energy, and do not wait for the leader to think for them.[15] One model (Figure 3-3) identifies 5 styles of followership[15]:

1. Passive
2. Conformist
3. Alienated
4. Pragmatic
5. Effective

Followers who emulate a *passive style* expect their leader to do their thinking for them, as well as to motivate them. *Conformists* are seen as the positive doers, but after they complete a delegated task, they still rely on their leader to tell them what is next. Alternatively, followers who tend to be *alienated* can think independently but exude negative energy. Often, these alienated followers are the ones who play the role of the devil's advocate, identifying all the reasons why a particular idea or plan will not work. *Pragmatic* followers are fence-sitters, or the ones who try to preserve the status quo and may eventually follow once enough people decide to do so. Followers who are the *effectives* can think for themselves, are very active, and exude positive energy.

A-HA! – WHAT IS YOUR FOLLOWERSHIP STYLE?

Refer to Figure 3-3 and plot yourself on the continuum of the y-axis (from independent critical thinker to dependent and not a critical thinker) and along the x-axis (from passive, not-engaged to actively engaged). Interpret your results.

As a follower, my style tends to be more like (circle one):

Passive   Conformist   Alienated   Pragmatic   Effective

Bottom Line!

"In the dance of leaders and followers, we change partners and roles throughout our lives. With each new partner, we must subtly adjust our movements and avoid the other's toes. If we are leading, we must lead; and if we are not, we must follow, but always as a strong partner."[17(p31)] – Ira Chaleff, Author, *The Courageous Follower*

Case Study: Personal Leadership Style— The Case of Elizabeth

As an emerging leader with limited experience, Elizabeth found that she could be influenced fairly easily by her peers and her supervisor. In most cases, she changed her style of interacting with others immediately after she received feedback from her supervisor or from her peers. For example, after her supervisor told her not to be so happy in the mornings, Elizabeth changed her approach to be more laid-back, even though it felt natural for her to arrive to the clinic with a smile on her face and a positive attitude, ready to start practicing. When Elizabeth was told that others perceived her to be aggressive and competitive, like a "puppy dog nipping at everyone's heels," she became a bit stumped. Elizabeth knew she was passionate and was comfortable with leading change, but had a hard time understanding how others could misinterpret her passion and enthusiasm as competitiveness or aggressiveness. And so, she toned down her passion and excitement about things in which she really cared, even though it didn't feel quite right. Elizabeth also realized that she struggled with leading other people because it was important for her to be liked. Therefore, she adapted her style when working with others to be more like them, even when it didn't feel comfortable. In one instance, Elizabeth became a bit more sarcastic when she worked closely with a peer who tended to be quite sarcastic and negative, so that she could relate better to this person's style.

However, Elizabeth started to recognize that this reactive, superficial approach to leadership was actually causing her to second-guess her ability to be an effective leader. She knew she was capable of building relationships with other people and in leading teams effectively, but as she flip-flopped her leadership style, Elizabeth started to feel less confident in making decisions and in her approach to connect with others. She realized that something was not working for her and that she needed to challenge her own understanding of leadership.

Elizabeth had always defined *leadership* as a role and as something she had to do. For example, as the team leader, Elizabeth knew that she had to direct or lead her team members to accomplish certain goals, by a certain timeframe, and, sometimes, in a certain way. However, what she discovered was that being a leader was something she had to be. She became intrigued to learn more about personal leadership, or leadership of self as an individual, and how to lead from the inside-out as a way to become an effective leader. She learned that she needed to fundamentally decide how she wanted to be, think, and perform—in ways in which she could leverage her passions and her strengths—to positively and authentically influence others.

Elizabeth discovered that developing her EQ was essential for effective leadership and was a good first step in her journey to develop her leadership style from the inside out. Increasing EQ required Elizabeth to take a sincere look at her core values, capabilities, passions, and strengths to become more intentional about her own development as a leader.

By becoming more self-aware through a process of self-assessment and self-reflection, Elizabeth discovered her strengths and her opportunities for personal change to strengthen her ability to influence, lead, and engage others in clinical practice. She noticed that she was able to initiate different responses once she changed how she interacted with others or how she approached situations. In other words, Elizabeth's ability to influence others as a leader and her ability to enhance team performance increased dramatically when she adapted and modified her own behavior first. Overall, by intentionally increasing her EQ, Elizabeth discovered that she was able to build stronger, more committed and engaged relationships because she learned how to connect with people better.

Chapter Key Words

Leadership Style, Classic Leadership Style, Authoritarian Leadership Style, Participative Leadership Style, Laissez-Faire Leadership Style, Charismatic Leadership Style, Quiet Leadership Style, Transactional Leadership Style, Situational Leadership Style, Servant Leadership Style, Transformational Leadership Style, Emotionally Intelligent Leadership Style, Followership, Extrovert, Introvert

References

1. Lewin K, Lippitt R, White RK. Patterns of aggressive behavior in experimentally created "social climates." *J Soc Psychol*. 1939;10(2):269-299.

2. Badaracco J. *Leading Quietly: An Unorthodox Guide to Doing the Right Thing*. Brighton, MA: Harvard Business Press; 2002.

3. Kahnweiler JB. *Quiet Influence: The Introvert's Guide to Making a Difference*. 1st ed. San Francisco, CA: Berrett-Koehler Publishers; 2013.

4. Cain S. *Quiet: The Power of Introverts in a World That Can't Stop Talking*. New York, NY: Broadway Books; 2013.

5. Hersey P. *The Situational Leader*. San Diego, CA: The Center for Leadership Studies; 1984.

6. Greenleaf Center for Servant Leadership. *What is Servant Leadership?* https://www.greenleaf.org/what-is-servant-leadership. Accessed September 28, 2018.

7. American Physical Therapy Association. *Professionalism in Physical Therapy: Core Values*. http://www.apta.org/Professionalism. Accessed March 21, 2020.

8. Burns JM. *Frank and Virginia Williams Collection of Lincolniana (Mississippi State University. Libraries). Leadership*. New York, NY: Harper & Row; 1979.

9. National Center for Healthcare Leadership. http://www.nchl.org. Accessed September 28, 2018.

10. Mark Langer. "Disney, Walt"; http://www.anb.org/articles/18/18-00309.html; American National Biography. Online Feb. 2000. Accessed March 21, 2020.

11. Kouzes JM, Posner BZ. *The Leadership Challenge: How to Make Extraordinary Things Happen in Organizations*. 6th ed. Somerset, NJ: John Wiley & Sons, Incorporated; 2017.

12. Goleman D. *Emotional Intelligence: Why It Can Matter More than IQ*. London, UK: Bloomsbury; 1996.

13. Goleman D. Leadership that gets results. *Harv Bus Rev*. 2000;78(2):4-17.

14. Skills You Need. *What Sort of Leader Are You?* http://www.skillsyouneed.com/ls/index.php/325444. Accessed October 22, 2018.

15. Kelley RE. *The Power of Followership: How to Create Leaders People Want to Follow, and Followers Who Lead Themselves*. New York, NY: Doubleday; 1992.

16. Latour SM, Rast VJ. Dynamic followership: The prerequisite for effective leadership. *Air Space Power J*. 2004;18(4):102.

17. Chaleff I. *The Courageous Follower: Standing up to & for Our Leaders*. 3rd ed. San Francisco, CA: Berrett-Koehler; 2009.

SUGGESTED READINGS

Hersey P. *The Situational Leader*. San Diego, CA: The Center for Leadership Studies; 1984.

Kahnweiler JB. *Quiet Influence: The Introvert's Guide to Making a Difference*. 1st ed. San Francisco, CA: Berrett-Koehler Publishers; 2013.

Kouzes JM, Posner BZ. *The Leadership Challenge: How to Make Extraordinary Things Happen in Organizations*. 6th ed. Somerset, NJ: John Wiley & Sons, Incorporated; 2017.

Learning to Lead Through Mentorship and Coaching

Jennifer Green-Wilson, PT, MBA, EdD

The growth and development of people is the highest calling of leadership.
— John C. Maxwell, American author, speaker, and pastor

CHAPTER OBJECTIVES

- Discuss the need for mentorship and coaching as it relates to leadership development.
- Examine characteristics for effective coaching.
- Examine characteristics for effective mentorship.
- Differentiate between mentorship and coaching.
- Self-assess your need for mentorship and coaching.

Green-Wilson J, Zeigler S, eds.
Learning to Lead in Physical Therapy (pp 57-72).
© 2020 Taylor & Francis Group.

Leadership Vignette

Angela M. Phillips, PT

One of my earliest mentors provided frequent opportunities for me to grow my skills in different ways. He taught, guided, and encouraged me, and provided insight and encouragement along the way. From this mentor, I learned how important it is to provide challenges and opportunities to individuals when you see potential and talent, and to invest in people. I truly believe that we should have passion and purpose in our careers as physical therapists. Because of this, I am committed to helping others find their passion and purpose. As professionals, I also believe we should give back to our profession by helping to shape the future. The best way to do that is through mentoring.

Mentoring can take on many forms—what is important is that we continue to mentor throughout our careers. I mentor because I enjoy seeing and knowing that others have succeeded with my help. I mentor in different ways. For potential new professionals, I offer to assist with preparation for college and/or job placement. For others, I have email, text, or phone relationships in which we share ideas and thoughts about specific projects. For others still, I have spent a fair amount of time discussing career goals and options and working on specific plans.

My advice for new professionals is to acknowledge that you will have many mentors throughout your career. Take advantage of the offers that people make to help and support. Seek mentors! Find people you respect and ask them to serve as mentors for you. Ask other colleagues in the field for information about experts to contact if you do not know whom to select. Seek mentors outside your area of interest, expertise, or field because they can provide you with unique opportunities to broaden and strengthen your professional growth and learning.

THE NEED FOR MENTORSHIP AND COACHING

Physical therapists and physical therapist assistants are obligated to engage in lifelong learning and to participate in professional development seeking diverse methods, settings, and types of experiences for attaining new competencies. Professional development includes leadership development. Mentoring and coaching are dynamic approaches that may be used effectively to help you develop your leadership and many other professional practice skills. Individuals can grow, develop, and become more effective when they have a mentor or coach who understands their potential value; helps them acquire, shape, and hone their leadership skills; and communicates confidence in their leadership capacity.[1]

DIFFERENTIATING MENTORING AND COACHING

Often "mentor" and "coach" are used interchangeably, and the line delineating how mentors and coaches engage in mentoring and coaching is becoming increasingly less distinct. Both coaching and mentoring experiences can create a safe place for individuals to test out and practice new behaviors and skills, although the relationship and skills of each are different.

Mentoring

Mentoring is an ongoing, collaborative relationship between 2 individuals, one of whom tends to be more experienced or senior than the other. The experienced mentor helps the less-experienced individual (*mentee*) grow and develop personally and professionally. The mentors focus on guiding and monitoring the general development of their mentees; these longer-term relationships unfold and strengthen over time. The relationship between the mentee and the mentor is often viewed as a partnership and, through mentorship, mentees may become more self-aware and energized for ongoing "self-reflection, learning, and action, leading to professional role development and growth."[2(p 46)]

Mentors can provide mentees with professional assistance, including general guidance, access to opportunities, entry into organizational and professional networks, and, sometimes, sponsorship. Also, they may be able to provide their mentees with valuable psychosocial support, teach them about the complexities of organizational or professional environments, help them with shaping their professional identity, or be role models for appropriate professional behaviors.[3,4] For example, mentees may learn by observing how their mentors interact with people and groups, then asking why their mentors modified their behaviors or leadership style in different situations. Through this dynamic process, mentees may develop a greater social awareness as well as their own self-awareness.

Individuals who have a mentor, vs those who do not, gain advantages including enhanced self-esteem and confidence, enhanced role socialization, greater opportunities for promotion and advancement, increased job satisfaction, higher incomes, and a well-defined career plan.[2,5]

Coaching

Alternatively, *coaching* may be viewed more as a training or development process in which a coach helps an individual (*coachee*) focus on certain performance issues or needs. Ultimately, through the process of coaching, the coachee achieves a specific goal or certain level of personal or professional competence. For example, physical therapist students often view their Clinical Educators (also referred to as *Clinical Instructors*) as their coaches during their clinical education experiences. During each clinical learning experience, students meet with these coaches to review specific goals and expectations, receive formal written feedback on their performance at midterm and final, and exchange ongoing, informal feedback throughout the day, especially when specific help is needed.

Coaches create awareness by helping people interpret what they are hearing, seeing, or feeling in more meaningful ways. Coaches try to help their coachees take responsibility for their behaviors and, ultimately, their performance. This intentional and effective process explains why some organizations may assign formal coaches to individuals or teams to build specific bench strength or talent intentionally.[6] The coaching process relies on collaboration, and opportunities for coaching include times when performance feedback needs to be given, current skills and strengths need to be expanded and developed, or individuals and teams might need help overcoming obstacles or barriers to goals and objectives. Typical times for formal coaching include during performance evaluation and periods of (annual) goal-setting, while episodic feedback to motivate or correct performance can happen at unscheduled times.

Team members who gain enhanced or new skills can take on new tasks or more responsibility, ultimately increasing individual and collective productivity. Effective coaching can overcome performance problems, develop skills, strengthen interpersonal and professional communication, enhance strategic thinking, foster a positive work environment, and improve retention. Good coaching produces greater job satisfaction, higher motivation, and greater engagement, and it improves relationships among others.

Activity 4-1: Where Could You Use a Mentor or Coach?

Brainstorm a list of professional or leadership related tasks, skills, or competencies for which you could use some short-term, specific coaching (eg, improving manual therapy skills or communication skills).

_____

_____

_____

_____

_____

_____

Next, brainstorm a list of professional or leadership-related career directions for which you might consider mentorship (eg, moving up in the company while juggling a family, or deciding whether to consider a specialization, residency, or advanced degree for what you want to do with your career).

_____

_____

_____

_____

_____

_____

Bottom Line!

Coaching is a shorter-term relationship usually used for development of a specific area, task, or skill, whereas mentoring is advantageous for longer-term career advisement and guidance focused on development of the mentee as a person and professional. Learning to lead will be most effective by establishing and cultivating mentoring and coaching relationships appropriately.

ESTABLISHING MENTORING AND COACHING RELATIONSHIPS: CONSIDERING STYLES AND SKILLS

Styles of interacting with others may yield different results. Recall in Chapter 3, several leadership styles were discussed. Mentors and coaches also have different styles. Therefore, it is important for you as mentees and coachees to be selective in finding a mentor or coach who has a style that is helpful for you.

By the same token, the coach and the mentor need to possess the skills necessary to be effective in the right way. While coaches ideally would need to possess expert knowledge and skill with abilities of interest to the coachee, they also need to be effective teachers. While a mentee needs to feel safe enough to disclose sensitive information, reveal weaknesses or challenges, and discuss lack of skills or competence, a mentor needs to provide confidential, nonjudgmental, sensitive feedback and to inspire, instruct, nurture, and encourage the mentee. Skills are needed for these relationships on both sides.

Activity 4-2: Identifying a Coach

Using your **first list** from Activity 4-1, identify a person or people in your life who might serve as a coach for the tasks/activities upon which you wish to improve.

_____

Why do you feel this person would be a good coach for what you have listed?

_____

_____

_____

What ideal skill sets and style do you need from your coach to have an effective coach-coachee relationship with you? Why?

_____

_____

_____

Activity 4-3: Selecting a Mentor

Using your **second list** from Activity 4-1, identify a person or people in your life who might serve as a mentor.

_____

As a mentoring relationship is usually more in-depth and longer term, the process of selecting the right person for you may benefit from further thought. For this activity, take the person you identified as a potential mentor, and use the checklist in Table 4-1[2] to help you become more aware of what that person—as a potential mentor—can and cannot offer you. Note, the first 6 questions focus on the other person's leadership skills and role expertise; the last 5 questions relate to this person's ability to be an effective mentor.[2] If you answer "no" to any of the first 6 questions, reconsider your potential selection as a mentor. If necessary, repeat the process with a different potential mentor.

Activity 4-4: The Ask

So far, you have identified areas in which you would like to have a coach or mentor (Activity 4-1), and you have identified individuals who you feel have the skill set to be a good coach or mentor for you (Activities 4-2 and 4-3). Now it is time to initiate the process. Contact the individual whom you have in mind, tell that person of the skill you would like to develop or the direction you would like to head (Activity 4-1), and ask if the person would be willing to be a coach or a mentor, depending on which relationship you are seeking. Point out why you are choosing the person. If the person says "yes," then establish a date and time for your first formal communication. If the person says "no," then ask for a recommendation for another person who might be able to meet your needs. Okay—get ready, get set, ask!

TABLE 4-1. A Sample Checklist for Finding the Mentor Who Is Right for You!			
DESIRED CHARACTERISTIC	YES	NO	DO NOT KNOW
1. Does this person have the technical expertise or the knowledge and skills in the competencies that you need to develop?			
2. Is this person a transformational leader by action and by example?			
3. Does this person have the ability to guide, support, affirm, and teach you?			
4. Is this person respected (in the profession, or health care organization, or community)?			
5. Does this person have access to important organizational/professional information, and can this person help you direct attention on important issues?			
6. Does this person have different networks of influential people (ie, is this person well-connected)?			
7. Is this person willing to assist you to be visible, credible, and accepted by others (in the organization/community/profession)?			
8. Is this person willing to work collaboratively with you?			
9. Is this person willing to spend the time and energy required for the development of your relationship?			
10. Are you comfortable with this person and trust this person to hold confidentiality?			
11. Is this person able to provide you with constructive as well as positive feedback?			
12. Can this person help you identify what you need to learn and provide the structure for learning experiences?			

Reprinted with permission from Barker, AM, Sullivan DT, Emery MJ. *Leadership Competencies for Clinical Managers: The Renaissance of Transformational Leadership*. Sudbury, MA: Jones and Bartlett Publishers; 2006.

Making the Most of Mentoring and Coaching

Now that you have an appropriate mentor or coach, it is time to focus on the relationship and prepare to be an effective mentee or coachee. The first focus is on gaining knowledge about building the relationship, followed by tips for maximizing effectiveness and understanding the lifespan of mentoring and coaching relationships.

Building the Relationship

As with leadership, building solid relationships is essential to fostering self-discovery, growth, and change. This also applies to mentoring and coaching relationships. The following list includes a few ways you can use being a mentee or coachee to expedite your ability to build rapport successfully:

- Demonstrate a willingness to be influenced.
- Express and demonstrate a sincere, personal interest in the feedback your mentors or coaches give.
- Demonstrate body language that is open and that supports engagement and trust. Avoid body language that is defensive.
- Be present. Allow enough space and time for seeing, hearing, and saying; create and ensure a safe place in which to share vulnerabilities.
- Suspend judgment.

Authors Buckingham and Coffman[7] and Maxwell[1] have developed further guidance for mentees and coachees to foster the most effective relationships with their mentors and coaches, including:

- Do not be afraid to experiment by trying out behaviors and then monitoring the reactions to see if there is a difference in others as a result of the difference in your own behavior. Ask for feedback. Mentorship and coaching relationships are meant to be safe places in which to learn.
- *Really* listen with your full attention during your next one-on-one conversation. Make eye contact and observe body language. Reflect upon what is being said, especially feedback. Try to connect with the story that is being told. Identify the underlying message.
- Try not to view silence as a waste of time, and try not to fill the silence. Use silent moments as time to think about what you have just heard or what you want to say, rather than formulating your answers and questions while your mentor or coach is still talking.
- Practice letting go of your assumptions, and approach each new interaction from an appreciative and mindful point of view. This means that you need to practice starting each interaction from the perspective of what is working well (or the positives) vs what is not working (or the negatives). Be optimistic and open-minded, and look for possibilities.
- Be approachable. Share personal experiences, stories, and lessons learned openly and honestly with your mentors and coaches. A word of caution—try not to share too many, and not too often!
- Self-advocate for your inclusion within certain teams, networks, and other departments within your organization. Share your diverse networks with others.

A-HA! – BEHAVIORS AND CHARACTERISTICS

In Chapter 2, characteristics of effective leaders were identified as proactive, passionate, authentic, emotionally intelligent, relationship builders, trustworthy, credible, and future-oriented.

Do you see similarities in the behaviors for being an effective mentee/coachee with those of being an effective leader?

_____

_____

_____

At which of the mentee/coachee behaviors do you feel you are best?

_____

_____

_____

Which behaviors do you need to work on?

_____

_____

_____

In past experiences as a coachee or mentee, do you feel you could have done a better job in those roles? Why or why not, and in what way(s)?

_____

_____

_____

●————————————————

Bottom Line!

Working toward effectiveness as a mentee/coachee also builds your leadership effectiveness.

Relationship Effectiveness

While both coaching and mentoring require a solid and admirable relationship between both parties, the longer-term nature of mentoring relationships hinges even more so on the establishment of a helping connection that is unique, open, deep, and grounded in mutual trust, respect, and honest communication.[8,9] Relationship-building takes time, energy, attention, and skill, and each party plays a mutual leadership role for the greatest effectiveness.

A Paradigm Shift to Leading Up

In the past, a mentor was seen as an authority figure instead of a partner, and the mentor adopted more of a directing or telling style. In the new (and more effective) paradigm of mentorship, the mentee takes responsibility for the relationship and the process. This is supported by Zachary in her book, _The Mentor's Guide: Facilitating Effective Learning Relationships_, in which she advocates for _learning partnerships_, or mentorship that is learning-centered and grounded in adult learning principles.[10] This perspective of mentorship fundamentally changes how mentees and mentors engage.

Note that teaching others and learning by doing have the highest retention rates, rather than being a passive recipient of advisement or information. These findings support the potential value to be gained by individuals who actively engage in mentorship or coaching activities. Thus, the current perspective of mentorship moves mentees from passive receivers to active, self-directed partners who are engaged actively in their own learning experience. Ideally, this means that the mentee, not the mentor, is the initiator and key overseer of this relationship. While coaching relationships may be more coach-directed for specific tasks, the coachee should still strive to take a leadership approach for the best learning experience.

Essentially, both mentees and coaches need to lead up. _Leading up_ requires individuals to learn how to self-manage their emotions, time, priorities, energy, thinking, words, and personal life. It requires them to be prepared every time they _connect up_, demonstrate behaviors to earn their mentor's or coach's trust, understand their priorities, and adapt their own style to connect better with their mentor's or coach's style.[1]

One of Maxwell's principles for leading up is to be prepared every time you take your leader's time.[1] In this case, the same principle holds true for every time you take the time of your mentor or coach. A large aspect of this requires proactively planning for your mentor or coachee meetings in advance to ensure you gain as much from the experience as possible, and that you foster a meaningful relationship by directing your efforts toward the expertise of your mentor or coach. Now imagine that you have a mentor or a coach.

How will you best prepare for the first and subsequent meetings?

_____

_____

_____

What questions would be most beneficial for you to ask during the meeting?

_____

_____

_____

How will you design the meeting so that it is respectful of the time of each party?

_____

_____

_____

What elements might you build in that adapt to the preferred style of the mentor or coach?

_____

_____

_____

The Phases of Mentoring and Coaching Relationships

Awareness of the phases, or stages, of mentoring and coaching relationships is helpful in progressing the mentorship and coaching conversations and for building successful experiences. Due to the differences in timespan and in focus, these stages differ between mentoring and coaching.

Mentoring relationships progress through 4 predictable phases (Figure 4-1) including preparing, negotiating, enabling, and coming to closure.[10] Movement through these 4 phases usually follows a fluid cycle with some overlap.[10]

In the first phase, or the *Preparing* phase, each time a new mentoring relationship begins, both the mentee and mentor need to prepare individually and together to explore their own motivations, and identify areas for their own learning and development, as well as their readiness to be actively engaged in a mentorship relationship. Initial conversations set the tone for the relationship, and before moving forward, both the mentee and mentor need to assess fairly quickly if they have an ability to connect and work collaboratively.

Phase 2 is the *Negotiating* phase, or the business phase, in which the mentee and mentor come to agreement on learning goals, define the content, and identify the process of the relationship or how they will work most effectively together. Ideally, mentees and mentors establish a mutual

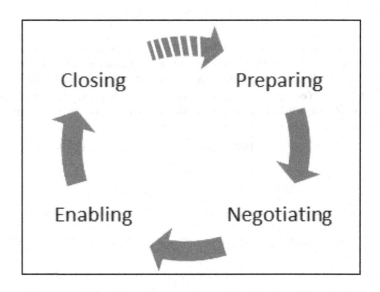

Figure 4-1. A model for mentoring. (Reprinted with permission from Zachary LJ. *The Mentor's Guide: Facilitating Effective Learning Relationships.* San Francisco, CA: Jossey-Bass, Inc.; 2000:51.)

understanding of assumptions, expectations, goals, needs, ground rules, confidentiality, boundaries, and limits, and hammer out logistics such as when to meet, how to meet, and how often.

Phase 3, or the *Enabling* phase, is the implementation phase, and it can be complex and long-lasting. Fundamentally, this phase requires the mentee and mentor to build and leverage effective communication skills, and to explore paths of connection, nurturing, learning, and development.

In Phase 4, or the *Closure* phase (which may or may not occur), the mentee and mentor may have the opportunity to evaluate their personal learning and growth experiences explicitly, and to acknowledging and celebrate achievements.

A-HA! – THE FOUR PHASES OF MENTORSHIP

Based on mentorship phases 1 and 2, describe the elements you will incorporate into your encounters to ensure they are successful.

_____

_____

_____

Look at the questions from "A-Ha! – Leading Up" on page 65. Learning from the 4 phases, how will you modify or add to what you already planned for your first and subsequent meetings with your mentor?

_____

_____

_____

What outcomes are you expecting from the relationship? What outcomes is your mentor expecting? (*Note*: Plan to have this discussion with your mentor at your first meeting.)

_____

_____

_____

Coaching also typically follows a phase process, although this may vary among the many types of coaching experiences. In health care, coaching can be formal or informal, and it includes professional, leadership, lifestyle, and executive coaching. While most coaching relationships are informal, formal organizational or professional coaching opportunities are also options. These relationships are usually timebound and conducted by an external and objective coach or consultant hired or brought in and assigned to an individual or group to deal with specific issues, skills, or situations. Like mentoring, coaching also usually follows a 4-stage process including awareness, analysis, action, and achievement.

In the awareness stage, the coach and coachee meet to discuss the coachee's background, expected goals, and outcomes. This meeting also helps establish the motivations of both the coach and coachee for the duration of the relationship.

In the second stage, analysis, the coach may have the coachee take some assessment to determine and understand the current level of the coachee's abilities. Reviewing these assessments will be one of the first steps taken to establish an action plan and to determine the frequency for coaching sessions.

The third stage is where the action and execution of specific changes are made. This may require the coachee to try new skills and behaviors, strengthen weaker areas, attend training sessions/programs, and implement other aspects from the analysis and action planning stages. Throughout this stage, the coach and coachee are in frequent contact, and revisions to the plan are discussed and modified as needed.

Finally, the achievement stage marks the time for feedback and review. It may involve reassessment of the coachees' skills compared to the start of the relationship, further attainment of feedback based on the assessment, and celebration of the outcomes. If the skill or task has been accomplished, this may be the end of the relationship, although, in the case of professional coaching, evidence shows that the best results are achieved when it is followed up with ongoing support through a mentor-like process. Therefore, the achievement phase is a good point for coachees to determine whether more could be gained by transitioning from the shorter-term coaching to the longer-term mentorship process.

A-HA! – REFLECTION ON COACHING

Think of a coaching relationship that you have had. It could be within sports, on-the-job coaching, or other forms.

Did the relationship include the 4 stages described in this section?

_____

_____

_____

What influence did you have within that relationship? Do you feel that you were an active or passive participant in gaining what you felt you needed from the relationship?

_____

_____

_____

What aspects within the stages of the coaching process do you feel you could have influenced more?

_____

_____

_____

When the relationship ended, did you consider where you wanted to go next with your newly developed skills?

_____

_____

_____

●———————————

Bottom Line!

Successful coaching and mentoring processes rely on frameworks that can be customized for maximum effectiveness, but that generally involve all stages of each process. Mentees and coachees should use knowledge of these frameworks to lead the way and gain the most from the relationships.

Fine-Tuning Through Reflection

Throughout both mentoring and coaching relationships, reflection is a key aspect and one of the ultimate benefits. Research indicates that adults learn and retain knowledge the best through consciously reflecting on their learning.[10] Reflection, considered as an introspective dialogue preferably carried on in written form, generates questions, provokes assessment of learning experiences, and enables the assimilation of new learning. In addition, during the mentoring process, reflecting "enables us to slow down, rest, and observe our journey and the process of self-knowledge that is so important along the way."[11(p57)] As a result , all participants will be in a better position to integrate their learning as well as derive meaning from the learning experiences.[10]

The process of reflection also fosters an awareness of individual factors that could potentially hinder the development of effective relationships, and then the chance to use strategies to work proactively toward overcoming these potential challenges. For example, it may be helpful for mentees to work on developing self-confidence or security in being vulnerable instead of feeling fearful about revealing a lack of skills or incompetence or feeling judged by others. As the relationship develops and unfolds, mentees may need to develop greater tolerance and patience for ambiguity, and courage and a willingness to change and adapt their own behaviors. Mentors, on the other hand, may need to practice facilitating others vs controlling, directing, telling, or being in charge.

A skill to be learned in the process of reflection is developing a comfort level with seeking, receiving, and using feedback. The development of expertise and mastery requires individuals to receive constructive, even critical feedback.[12] While most people realize that feedback is a necessary component of reflection and growth, they are often hesitant to make themselves vulnerable to it. Receiving feedback can be awkward, embarrassing, and sometimes, even hurtful, yet feedback is at the center of any learning process.[13] Basically, feedback is information about how people are doing in their efforts to reach a goal. Receiving feedback is the only way for individuals to know whether they are close to their goals or whether they are executing properly. Helpful feedback is goal-referenced, tangible, transparent, actionable, user-friendly (specific and personalized), timely, ongoing, and consistent.[14] Mentees and coachees should participate in the process of gaining helpful feedback along the way as their relationships develop.

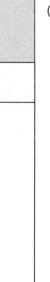

TABLE 4-2. EFFECTIVE MENTORING AND COACHING QUESTIONS WORKSHEET			
TYPE OF QUESTION	**DESCRIPTION**	**GENERAL EXAMPLES**	**YOUR EXAMPLES**
Open-ended questions	Invite participation, disclosure, and commitment	"Have you tried _____?" "What do you think is the best way to _____?" "What do you think would happen if you _____?" "Tell me more about _____." "What are you going to do next?"	
Discovery questions	Promote self-discovery	"What's new or different?" "What's the gap?" "What's *really* going on?"	
Questions used to assess knowledge and understanding	Reveal an individual's or team's understanding of reality, challenges, and performance strengths and gaps	"What do you see as the biggest challenge?" "What will it take to address the challenge?" "What are our strengths?" "Where are the gaps in skills, attitudes, or behaviors?"	

(continued)

Activity 4-5: Seeking Feedback

Mentees and coachees (as well as mentors and coaches) can benefit from practicing how to ask questions effectively and how or when to use different types of questions for obtaining feedback. Many of these types of questions are provided with examples in this section.

Plan to seek feedback from your encounters with your coach or mentor that you have selected earlier in this chapter. In Table 4-2, write in sample questions that you could use for your process to seek feedback from your coach or mentor.

Bottom Line!

Reflection is a vital part of effective relationship building and in learning to lead. Developing and implementing the skill of obtaining and responding effectively to feedback is necessary for accelerating the growth process in all areas of your life.

TABLE 4-2 (CONTINUED). EFFECTIVE MENTORING AND CONTINUED COACHING QUESTIONS WORKSHEET			
TYPE OF QUESTION	**DESCRIPTION**	**GENERAL EXAMPLES**	**YOUR EXAMPLES**
Questions to determine readiness and motivation	Reveal the current state of action and level of engagement	"Are you ready?" "*When* will you be ready?" "What are you most excited about?" "What's holding you back?"	
Clarifying questions	Elucidate current situation, problem, need, challenge, or goal, or reveal personal feelings, concerns, questions, or anxieties	"What do the data reveal about the situation?" "How do you feel about this?"	
Stimulating questions	Capture current fundamental opportunity, foster a search for shared meaning, or create a new or changed framework	"What is the opportunity underlying this challenge?" "What are you/we not doing/paying attention to that would completely shift this situation?" "What are you/we not talking about that you/we should be talking about to solve this problem/seize this opportunity?" "If all constraints were removed, what courses of action would be available to you or the team?"	
Forwarding action questions	Move the individual or team forward	"What steps are necessary to move the task/project forward?" "Who else needs to be involved to ensure success?" "What obstacles need to be eliminated?"	

Reprinted with permission from Goleman, D. Leadership That Gets Results. *Harv Bus Rev*, March-April 2000:78-90.

Case Study: Mentoring, Coaching, and Reflection

When Tom started his first assignment as a formal leader in a physical therapist practice, he knew he needed to seek the help of a mentor and a coach. He needed a mentor to guide him in setting his personal and professional goals and in drafting his professional development plan. He also needed a coach to help him be successful in this particular, formal leadership position, since it was a new role for him. Because of these different needs, Tom decided that it would be valuable to work with 2 individuals because he understood that mentorship and coaching were different interactions that could yield different results. He recognized that it was his responsibility, as the mentee and coachee, to initiate these relationships by asking each person for assistance.

Fortunately, Tom found a knowledgeable coach who helped to clarify specific role expectations and responsibilities, and how to become socialized to the culture of his department and the organization. The coaching sessions were pre-planned, and held weekly for the first 6 months. Tom came prepared to each meeting with questions he needed answered.

As it turned out, Tom's mentor found him! This person invited Tom to lunch and, during the meal, asked Tom a sequence of reflective questions to help him establish a few key long-term professional goals. Throughout this dialogue, Tom's mentor also helped him navigate through decision-making pathways within the organization to assist him in his current role, and invited him to a couple of networking events so that Tom could become more comfortable working with executives on the senior management team.

Often, Tom was told by his immediate supervisor and his coach that he was exceeding performance expectations and that many on the executive leadership team noticed his strong performance. Tom felt comfortable knowing that he had a coach and a mentor helping him, especially for when new leadership opportunities opened up, because he wanted to continue to learn and grow as a leader and to move up within the organization. He thought he was well-positioned for his next promotion. Yet over time, Tom became confused when he noticed that he was being passed over for promotions. Upon reflection, Tom decided that he had to act.

Tom approached his manager, who was also one of his mentors, to inquire as to why he had not been considered for the promotions. He was shocked when his manager told him that he had been identified as a possible candidate for both promotions, but because the leadership team perceived Tom to be happy and content in his current leadership position, they decided to keep him in his role so that he could keep performing well for the organization. After receiving this feedback, Tom realized that he needed to be much more open, intentional, and honest about his long-term goals for career advancement, and that he needed to explicitly ask his manager/mentor to be an advocate for him the next time a promotion was available. Tom also realized that he needed to be more proactive and assert himself in initiating and following up on conversations with his mentor to create greater clarity about his professional goals.

CHAPTER KEY WORDS

Mentor, Mentee, Coaching, Coachee, Reflection

References

1.   Maxwell JC. *The 360 Degree Leader: Developing Your Influence from Anywhere in the Organization.* Nashville, TN: Thomas Nelson, Inc.; 2005.

2.   Barker AM, Sullivan DT, Emery MJ. *Leadership Competencies for Clinical Managers: The Renaissance of Transformational Leadership.* Sudbury, MA: Jones and Bartlett; 2006.

3.   Roemer L. Women CEOs in health care: did they have mentors? *Health Care Manage Rev.* 2002;27(4):57-67.

4.   Walsh AM, Borkowski SC, Reuben EB. Mentoring in health administration: the critical link in executive development/practitioner application. *J Healthc Manag.* 1999;44(4):269.

5.   Grindel CG. Mentoring managers. *Nephrol Nurs J.* 2003;30(5):517.

6.   Cheese P, Thomas RJ, Craig E. *The Talent Powered Organization: Strategies for Globalization, Talent Management, and High Performance.* London, UK; Kogan Page; 2008.

7.   Buckingham M, Coffman C. *First, Break All the Rules: What the World's Greatest Managers Do Differently.* New York, NY: Simon & Schuster; 1999.

8.   Vance C. Mentoring at the edge of chaos. *Nurse Lead.* 2003;1(1):42-43.

9.   Klein E, Dickerson-Hazzard N. Reflections on nursing leadership. *Reflect Nurs Leadersh.* 2000;26(3):18-22.

10. Zachary LJ. *The Mentor's Guide: Facilitating Effective Learning Relationships.* 1st ed. San Francisco, CA: Jossey-Bass Publishers; 2000.

11. Huang CA, Lynch J. *Mentoring: The Tao of Giving & Receiving Wisdom.* New York, NY: Harper Collins Publishers; 1995.

12. Ericsson KA, Prietula MJ, Cokely ET. The making of an expert. *Harv Bus Rev.* 2007;85(7/8):114.

13. Kouzes JM, Posner BZ. *The Leadership Challenge: How to Make Extraordinary Things Happen in Organizations.* 6th ed. Somerset, NJ: John Wiley & Sons, Incorporated; 2017.

14. Wiggins G. Seven keys to effective feedback. *Educ Leadersh.* 2012;70(1):10-16.

Suggested Readings

Maxwell JC. *The 360 Degree Leader: Developing Your Influence From Anywhere in the Organization.* Nashville, TN: Thomas Nelson, Inc.; 2005.

Zachary LJ. *The Mentor's Guide: Facilitating Effective Learning Relationships.* 1st ed. San Francisco, CA: Jossey-Bass Publishers; 2000.

UNIT 2

LEADING OTHERS AS A POSITIVE INFLUENCE

As you learn to lead, you will continue to discover that being a leader means leveraging your social influence to lead others in multiple directions—down, up, across, and out. You can lead—influence others—from anywhere, as informal or personal leaders, and you do not need to be in a formal leadership role to lead. In this book, leadership is about action and behavior—what leaders do. From this lens, the leader uses certain behaviors intentionally to influence a group of individuals to act. By building and influencing these dynamic relationships, you will achieve shared goals at all levels of practice.

Collaboration, teamwork, and communication can affect patients and patient outcomes positively. Individuals who are collaborative are described as cooperative, and cooperation happens when a mutually beneficial exchange takes place between 2 or more entities—even if their ideas are different. Collaboration happens when people cooperate willingly instead of competing. Collaboration and cooperation require an abundance mindset that focuses on the win-win, believes there is enough for everyone, and understands that more can be achieved together.

However, without an explicit set of expectations about what it means to work collaboratively with others or how collaboration should look in terms of behaviors, individuals may have to use their own interpretation of collaboration. Therefore, it makes sense to proactively clarify the mindset that collaborative individuals need to bring to their team and to their work, the abilities and skills they need to master while working in teams, and the personal leadership and communication styles that work well in diverse team environments. Additionally, it is critical that team leaders role model and demonstrate the collaborative behaviors they want their team members to mirror.

In this unit, emphasis is on exploring how you can lead as a collaborative member of any group. Recall that leadership styles vary from person to person, and some leadership styles are more effective than others, especially at engaging and inspiring teams to action. Over the next 4 chapters, you will start to discover how you tend to communicate, cooperate, assert yourself, and collaborate as an individual on any team. You will be provided with some ideas on how you can lead as a member of a group, how to continue to build your own leadership capacity by embracing inclusive and diverse teamwork, and why this makes a difference.

5

Communicating Effectively
Using the Language of Leadership

Jennifer Green-Wilson, PT, MBA, EdD

People cannot succeed in life without communicating effectively.
It's not enough just to work hard or to do a great job. To be successful,
you need to learn how to really communicate with others.
— *John C. Maxwell, American author, speaker, and pastor*

CHAPTER OBJECTIVES

- Examine the key elements of effective communication.
- Discuss why effective leadership requires effective communication skills.
- Self-assess your communication style.
- Describe how listening can influence communication.
- Discuss how storytelling and leadership are related.
- Identify 2 ways in which you can adapt your communication style to strengthen your effectiveness at communicating.

Green-Wilson J, Zeigler S, eds.
Learning to Lead in Physical Therapy (pp 75-92).
© 2020 Taylor & Francis Group.

Leadership Vignette

Karen Mueller, PT, DPT, PhD

My beliefs about the importance of communication took shape in adolescence as I became interested in the work of my psychiatrist father. Through our discussions, I began to recognize the compelling relationship between psychological distress and poor communication at the intrapersonal or interpersonal levels. My father's examples ignited a lifelong interest in exploring the development of effective communication as an instrumental skill for optimal wellbeing, even superseding intellectual capacity. As an example, I recall a physical therapy school classmate with a 4.0 GPA who subsequently failed an internship because of an abrasive communication style. When I became the Academic Coordinator of Clinical Education in the physical therapy program at Northern Arizona University, I saw this pattern repeat: students rarely failed because of poor clinical skills; instead, the problems most often resided in the failure to communicate appropriately. Because I was also teaching the communication courses, I felt the need to explicitly demonstrate the value (and science) of effective professional communication, which led to my writing a book on the topic.

My passion for teaching and writing about effective communication stems from my belief that interactive excellence is the most important skill for personal and professional self-actualization. In the personal realm, the ability to build and sustain satisfying relationships has long been recognized as beneficial for emotional and psychological health during life's challenges. In the professional realm, effective communication builds collegial relationships that nurture and sustain us. I have learned that solid work relationships allow us to create change together and enhance career satisfaction. Physical therapy intervention is provided in the context of the therapeutic alliance, which is grounded in authentic, compassionate communication. Therefore, our patients need to know we care about them as people before they care about what we can offer them as professionals.

I have also learned that, unfortunately, in the absence of ensuring accurate self-reflection and mindful self-awareness (intrapersonal communication skills), developing social and emotional intelligence (interpersonal communication skills), or negotiating consensus-driven change (an instrumental communication skill), the odds of alienating patients, colleagues, and other team members are substantial, particularly if the offender has somehow found a way into a leadership role. Working with such an individual can lead to resentment, frustration, and burnout. Thus, I believe that skills for an effective leader are in the 3 main areas of communication: with self, with others, and with organizations. Technology has increased the complexity of each of these areas as it encourages limited nonverbal communication, which creates opportunity for misunderstanding or frank misuse (eg, a colleague fired by email).

The physical therapy profession, like all health care disciplines, faces considerable challenges in the midst of health care reform, and the need for effective communication skills has never been greater. To improve our communication, we must first value it (just as our patients must be motivated to adhere to their plan of care). Once motivated, I believe that practicing mindfulness through daily meditation (which is the essence of intrapersonal communication) is crucial for developing the self-awareness and the beginner's mindset needed for addressing what we know, and being honest with ourselves in what we do not know. With mindfulness, transitioning to emotionally intelligent interpersonal communication becomes more seamless, as does the ability to lead others through consensus.

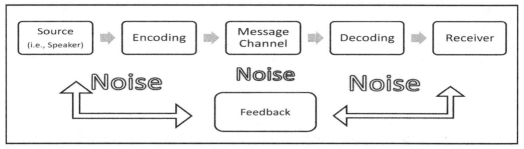

Figure 5-1. Traditional communication model. (Adapted from Shannon CE, Weaver W. *The Mathematical Theory of Communication*. Urbana, IL: University of Illinois Press; 1949.)

Box 5-1

ELEMENTS OF AUTHENTIC AND COLLABORATIVE CONVERSATIONS

- Ask questions: Stimulate a different level of discussion and engagement by asking open-ended questions to explore what others think.
- Level with people: Show people where you stand, and say what you think and feel. Show that you are open to considering alternative views. Ensure there are no hidden agendas, and confront tough issues.
- Show vulnerability: Build trust and feel comfortable saying, "I don't know"; "I was wrong"; or "I need help."
- Build on the inputs of others: Listen carefully; use "yes, and" rather than "yes, but."
- Share stories: Understand that listeners may listen successfully to a story to gain the essence of an experience; they do not need to accept or reject the story because a "story is a story."
- Encourage others to share their stories: Realize that sharing stories needs to go both ways; everyone gains more information about each other through exchanging stories.

Reprinted with permission from Denning S. *The Secret Language of Leadership.* San Francisco, CA: John Wiley & Sons, Inc.; 2007:203-204.

COMMUNICATION AND LEADERSHIP

Communication is the process of sending and receiving information between people. Effective communication is not as easy to achieve as it would seem, given the plentiful opportunities for noise to interrupt and potentially disrupt the process (Figure 5-1).[1] Effective communication requires the sender and the receiver to deliver a message that is clear and translated well. Feedback is important to ensure that the right message is received, or to clarify if the message is or is not understood.

Useful communication needs to be a conversation or a dialogue, not a monologue. A dialogue can be an informal conversation, formal discussion, or negotiation between two or more people about opinions, ideas, feelings, or routine issues, and sometimes about opposing perspectives. Ideally, dialogues need to be collaborative and, in a productive one, people listen to each other to find common ground, meaning, and mutual agreement. Those who lead can facilitate more collaborative conversations by asking questions, leveling with people, showing vulnerability, sharing authentic stories, and encouraging others to share their stories (Box 5-1).[2]

Leadership communication is about influencing others: setting mutual goals, changing perspectives, changing behavior, and inducing action. When leaders who are learning to lead focus on developing their influencing skills, they also enhance their ability to share information, persuade, negotiate, and connect with others. This chapter will focus on improving effectiveness in communication and, subsequently, leadership capacity.

Bottom Line!

"Leadership is about communication." – Daniel Goleman, author and science journalist

BASIC COMMUNICATION STYLES

Many communication styles can and should be used to demonstrate effective leadership, and the style used depends on the audience, message, and desired effect. An effective communication style is a mixture of verbal communication, nonverbal communication (ie, body language), and listening.

Verbal Communication

Individuals who use effective verbal communication skills employ spoken words that are readily understood by others, and they express their words with appropriate enunciation, emphasis, and tone of voice. The basic verbal communication approaches are passive, assertive, aggressive, passive-aggressive, and persuasive (Table 5-1).[3] How these methods are used may impact not only the transfer of information, but also the ability to connect and form effective relationships.

Activity 5-1: Your Verbal Communication Approach

1. Review Table 5-1 in which the communication styles are described.
2. Select the style that seems to describe your most typical approach to communication. Try to make your choice as spontaneously as possible; in other words, do not overanalyze your decision.
3. Identify the style that seems the least typical of your approach to communication, and reflect on why you made this decision.
4. Have several trusted people look at the list and tell you what they think your most typical and least typical approaches to verbal communication are. Does the feedback match your self-assessment? Consider why or why not.

Ideally, leaders learning to lead need to model an assertive communication style because this style is the one that is the most effective for building and maintaining effective, mutually respectful relationships. Individuals using assertive communication styles are able to state their opinions and feelings clearly and directly, as well as advocate firmly for their needs without infringing upon anyone else.

Nonverbal Communication

Nonverbal communication incorporates behaviors such as gestures, facial expressions, body posture, the proximity to the listener, eye contact, dress, and appearance. Nonverbal communication also includes other aspects of speech (distinct from words) that transmit meaning, including pitch, speed, tone, and volume of voice.

Envision that one of your peers stomps into your clinical office area, throws a patient's chart onto the desk, flops dramatically down in a chair, and then looks straight ahead at a bare wall. Eventually,

TABLE 5-1. VERBAL COMMUNICATION STYLES	
COMMUNICATION STYLE	**DESCRIPTION/CHARACTERISTICS**
Passive	Neglects to express your feelings, needs, or opinions
	Neglects to defend your viewpoints
	Exhibits poor eye contact and submissive body posture
	Speaks softly or apologetically
Aggressive	May use "you" statements and not "I" statements; for example, "Why did you do that? You know better than to do that."
	May speak in a loud, demanding, and overbearing voice with piercing eye contact and an arrogant body posture
	May not listen well, and may interrupt frequently
	May criticize, blame, or confront others
Passive-Aggressive	May deny there is a problem
	May mutter to yourself under your breath rather than confront the person or issue
	May have difficulty acknowledging your anger
	May use facial expressions that do not match how you feel (ie, smiling when angry)
Assertive	Able to express needs, wants, and feelings clearly, appropriately, and respectfully
	Listens well without interrupting
	Uses good eye contact and has a relaxed body posture
	Speaks in a calm and clear tone of voice
	Connects with others
Reprinted with permission from Youker, Robert. Using the Communications Styles Instrument for Teambuilding. *Proj Manag World J.* 2013;II(VII). https://pmworldjournal.com. Accessed October 7, 2018.	

someone asks, "Is everything okay?" but the, "I'm fine" response is said in a curt tone with no eye contact. In this scenario, most people would pay more attention to the message sent via nonverbal communication (eg, lack of eye contact and verbal tone) rather than the actual words spoken.[4] Research suggests that nonverbal messages are believed more so than the verbal ones, especially when the message is asymmetric, meaning that the nonverbal message is incongruent with the verbal one.[4] In general, experts indicate that between 50% and 80% of all communication is nonverbal, and that nonverbal communication carries between 65% and 93% more impact than the actual words spoken, especially when messages involve emotional meaning and attitudes.[4]

Effective and carefully selected nonverbal communication is critical for effective leadership. Nonverbal cues may be exchanged rapidly in a face-to-face interaction.[5] Body language, in particular, is meaningful especially when a person meets someone for the first time. Therefore, leaders learning to lead need to be aware that body language may be very influential in forming first impressions. The face, eyes, and hands are particularly influential parts of the body in sending nonverbal or body language signals. In fact, universal facial expressions for happiness, sadness, fear, disgust, surprise, and anger have been identified that convey human emotion in the same way across cultures. Eyes are also part of facial expressions and are important as they can convey massive feeling in a particular glance with no words spoken. Finally, hands and arms may be used to convey messages through pointing; drawing in the air; conveying common signals such as OK, thumbs-up, victory-sign, or possibly inappropriate gestures; and to greet people "hello" or wave "goodbye." Arms may send a defensive signal when crossed in front of the body and, conversely, indicate feelings of openness and safety when held at a person's side, with palms up and open.

Nonverbal communication can make or break a leader's speech. If the leader is trying to inspire yet has poor body language and speaks with a monotone voice, then the audience may not receive the message as inspirational. Thus, developing an awareness to read body language and to understand the messages being sent through body language helps leaders become much more effective in their ability to communicate.

Activity 5-2: Video Your Communication

1. Step 1: Video yourself in normal conversation, giving a presentation, or any other scenario of communication. Review the video at least once, and jot down verbal and nonverbal communication behaviors that you demonstrated.

2. Step 2: Assess the effectiveness of your demonstrated verbal and nonverbal communication skills relative to scope and context of presentation topic. Do you feel that your nonverbals were effective? Why or why not?

Listening

Listening is the third required communication skill for effective leadership, and this skill can dramatically impact a leader's ability to influence and connect with others. Unfortunately, and often, people appear to be going through the motions of listening and, in reality, just take turns speaking but do not really or sincerely listen to what others say. Therefore, it is important to differentiate hearing from listening.

Hearing is a physical ability, one of your 5 senses, while listening is a skill that can be developed. It is both possible to hear but not listen, and to listen but not hear. For example, someone who can physically hear may actually be a poor listener, while people who are hearing-impaired may be good listeners because they pay closer attention to all of the information being conveyed.

Regardless, poor listening always limits interpersonal communication, so it is imperative for both the sender and receiver to work on developing listening skills and then seek feedback regarding perceptions of the ability to listen. In the long run, developing the ability to listen takes effort, energy, and work.

Activity 5-3: Stop Talking and Listen!

Ask a peer for help! Tell a colleague that you want to work on *really* listening to others, and ask for feedback. Listen for input as to how you make others feel when you are practicing good listening skills.

If you perform Activity 5-3 with enough people, you may identify some themes or your types (styles) of listening. Multiple sources have described types of listening, including[6-8]:

- Passive listening, or not listening: Completely ignoring the speaker, multitasking (ie, texting someone else when another person is talking to you face-to-face)
- Pretend or semi-responsive listening: Using behaviors or responses (ie, routine nods, fake smiles, saying "uh-huh" and "of course") to demonstrate an appearance of listening
- Biased or selective listening: Intentionally picking and choosing what information is heard, and possibly disregarding or dismissing certain viewpoints

- Misinterpreted listening: Unconsciously overlaying your own interpretations of the information received, or possibly trying to make certain pieces of information fit in the conversation where they do not
- Active or attentive listening: Expending energy and effort in the process of listening, possibly to gather certain information for your own purposes
- Engaged listening: Asking open-ended questions and probing to clarify or enhance information received
- Empathic listening: Sincerely and deeply trying to understand the other person's perspective, and frequently testing facts as well as feelings throughout the dialogue. The essence of empathic listening is not to agree with someone, but rather to fully and deeply understand the other person both emotionally and intellectually.

A-HA! – WHAT TYPE OF LISTENER ARE YOU?

Now that you have read about types of listening, use the feedback from having done Activity 5-3 to answer the following questions:

What kind of listener do you tend to be?

_____

_____

What type of listener do you want to be? Why?

_____

_____

What could you practice to become your desired type of listener?

_____

_____

How would these changes impact your skill as a listener?

_____

_____

Bottom Line!

"The single biggest problem in communication is the illusion that it has taken place."
– George Bernard Shaw, Irish playwright, critic, polemicist, and political activist

COMMUNICATION STYLES

Just as there are different styles of leadership, discussed in Chapter 3, there are also different styles of communicating that can affect the ability to lead effectively. One way to understand your style of communication is by noticing where you fall on a continuum. Covey uses a continuum model that moves from dependence to independence to interdependence to describe personal and interpersonal development through language.[6] Specifically, Covey defines:

- Dependence as the "you" paradigm: Dependent people need others to get what they need or want (eg, "You need to get me that article so that I can read it before class.").
- Independence as the "I" paradigm: Independent people can get what they want through their own effort (eg, "I am able to access the article that I need to read for class.").
- Interdependence as the "we" paradigm: Interdependent people combine their efforts to achieve greater success (eg, "Let's see what we can uncover about the topic discussed in this article. Let's compare our findings together.").

A-HA! – VIDEO REVISITED

Review the videotape you took of yourself communicating in Activity 5-2.

How many statements did you make reflecting dependence, independence, and interdependence development approaches?

_____

_____

How many nonverbal behaviors did you display that communicated each?

_____

_____

Was that your intention in your communication? Why or why not?

_____

_____

A more concrete method for understanding your communication style is through the Social Style Model developed by the 1964 work of Dr. David W. Merrill, an industrial psychologist and university professor who started researching predictors of success in management. His work formed the foundation of the Social Style Model as well as the start-up of the TRACOM Group.[9] Through his research, Merrill discovered that people tend to demonstrate consistent, observable behaviors, and that others agreed consistently on certain words used to describe each of these behaviors. The concept of social style is helpful in categorizing how people interact with others interpersonally, and the model developed by the TRACOM Group provides insight into verbal and nonverbal communication tendencies based on social style (Figure 5-2).[9]

In Figure 5-2, on the vertical axis, notice the 2 opposing dimensions as controls (top) and emotes, or shows emotions (bottom), which measure assertiveness; and, on the horizontal axis, the 2 opposing dimensions, tells (left) and asks (right), measure how responsive or vocal someone is to different experiences. Using this framework to combine dimensions, 4 distinct social styles with unique communication characteristics become apparent. They are summarized here and detailed in Table 5-29:

1. Analytical style (controls and asks): Characterized by a process-oriented communication style
2. Driver style (controls and tells): Characterized by a direct and action-oriented communication style
3. Expressive style (emotes and tells): Characterized by an idea-oriented style
4. Amiable style (emotes and asks): Characterized by a people-oriented communication style

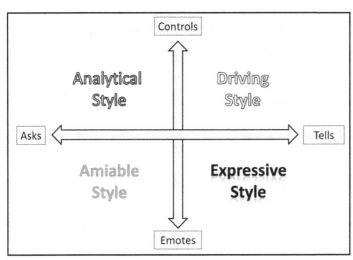

Figure 5-2. The Social Style Model impacting communication styles. (Adapted from Social Style Model Overview & Style Descriptions. The TRACOM Group. Available at: http://www.tracomcorp.com/training-products/model/style-descriptions.html. Accessed September 8, 2018.)

TABLE 5-2. AN OVERVIEW OF FOUR SOCIAL STYLES IMPACTING COMMUNICATION STYLES

STYLE DESCRIPTION	APPROACH TO DECISION MAKING	TIME ORIENTATION
Analytical Style		
Values facts, accuracy, competency, and logic over opinions Described by others as quiet, logical, sometimes reserved May appear distant from others, uncommunicative, and independent May not communicate with others unless there is a specific need to do so May avoid risk and favors cautious, deliberate decisions	Tends to make decisions based on facts and verifiable data; needs evidence	Moves with deliberateness; takes time to review all facts and available data Has strong time discipline combined with slow pace to action Does not respond well to being rushed
Driver Style		
May be seen by others as active, forceful, and determined; direct Initiates social interaction; focuses efforts on goals and objectives to be accomplished Wants to know estimated outcome of each option May be willing to accept risks, but wants to move quickly and have the final say Tends to focus on efficiency or productivity rather than relationships	Prefers facts, useful information, and viable options Does not like being told what to do	Prefers getting to the point, staying on target Prefers sticking to "the schedule" Not tolerant of actions if deemed a waste of time

(continued)

TABLE 5-2 (CONTINUED). AN OVERVIEW OF FOUR SOCIAL STYLES IMPACTING COMMUNICATION STYLES		
STYLE DESCRIPTION	**APPROACH TO DECISION MAKING**	**TIME ORIENTATION**
Expressive Style		
Openly displays positive and negative feelings May appear reactive or spontaneous Personable, talkative, may sometimes be opinionated Moves quickly, continually excited about the "next big idea" Enjoys taking risks	Risk-taker based on opinions of others May value opinions more than facts	Tends to act quickly and not be disciplined about time May change course rapidly
Amiable Style		
People-oriented; cares about relationships more so than results or tasks Effective at achieving rapport with others Usually appears warm, friendly, and cooperative	Often uses personal opinions and feelings to arrive at decisions Prefers to avoid direct confrontations Values input of others; decision-making process can be influenced by others Not a risk-taker; attempts to reduce risk by ensuring actions will not damage relationships	Tends to move slowly, and is not disciplined about time Needs/wants time for small talk and socializing before moving to any specific issue or work
Reprinted with permission from Social Style Model Overview & Style Descriptions. The TRACOM Group. https://tracom.com/social-style-training. Accessed March 21, 2020.		

Activity 5-4: Social Style Self-Assessment

Review the styles from Table 5-2. What Social Style do you think you exhibit? Why?

_____

_____

Bottom Line!

Understanding your own communication and social styles and another person's communication and social styles will help you, as a leader learning to lead, become a more effective communicator because you will understand how styles interact well together and which styles may inherently cause communication problems.

EFFECTIVENESS IN COMMUNICATING

Many sources of misunderstanding can impact communication, and it is important to appreciate that each person has a different context or life experience associated with each word and gesture used while communicating. Frequently, what one person means by a particular word or action may mean something different to another. Also, if words and actions contradict each other, people may pay closer attention to the actions and, ultimately, may miss important meanings in the verbalized message. Reacting emotionally or being in an emotional state may also inhibit the ability of the speaker or the receiver to connect while communicating. Fortunately, you can modify or change your behaviors to enhance your own interpersonal communication. Methods discussed in this section include adapting your communication style, being an effective storyteller, developing the art of persuasion, and mastering written and technologic strategies of communication.

Adapting Your Communication Style

It is important for you, as a leader learning to lead, to self-manage your own communication style and to know how to adjust your own approach to become more effective when communicating with others. For example, using the Social Styles model just discussed in Table 5-2, the following tips show how to adjust your communication accordingly for greatest success[9]:

- Analytical style: If the other person's style of communication tends to be more analytical (process-oriented), then you:
  - Outline your proposal (1, 2, 3…) in a logical, precise order.
  - Break down the recommendations and include options with pros and cons for each recommendation.
- Driver style: If the other person's style of communication tends to be more of a driver (action-oriented) style, then you:
  - Focus on the results and state the conclusion at the beginning of the conversation.
  - State your best recommendation, and do not offer too many alternatives.
  - Be brief, and emphasize the practicality of your ideas.
- Expressive style: If the other person's style of communication tends to be more expressive (idea-oriented), then you:
  - Be conceptual; start with the big picture and work toward the specific details.
  - Allow enough time for discussion.
  - Do not get impatient when the individual goes off on tangents.
- Amiable style: If the other person's style of communication tends to be more amiable (people-oriented), then you:
  - Allow time for informal, small talk; do not start the formal discussion right away.
  - Stress the relationships between your proposal and the people concerned.

Activity 5-5: Adapting Your Style

Through observation, identify people you know who have each of these communication/social styles. Practice a plan for adapting your communication to each person's style during your next encounter. Execute your plan with at least one of those people today!

Gaining Clarity Through Storytelling

As you learned in Chapter 1, storytelling is an essential communication skill for leaders because stories can be tailored and personalized to meet different needs in many situations. Storytelling can help leaders be effective communicators when they need to inspire an individual, team, or organization to look toward the future. It can also help when leaders need to establish a shared vision to spark change, impart lessons, share knowledge, define culture and transmit values, and explain who they are and what they believe.[2] Leaders can establish credibility and authenticity through telling their real-world stories. When leaders believe deeply in their stories, they can have an impact and inspire creativity, engagement, and transformation. However, as a leader learning to lead by using storytelling, you need to plan and prepare carefully for it to be useful; winging it might not be enough, and this approach could backfire.[2]

Activity 5-6: A Powerful Story

A great example of how leaders can use storytelling to change minds and actions came during the discussion about the new vision for the profession of physical therapy in the American Physical Therapy Association 2013 House of Delegates. California delegate Terrence M. Nordstrom was instrumental in defining the human experience through his storytelling. A video clip of Dr. Nordstrom's story may be accessed at: http://www.apta.org/Vision/HumanExperience. By listening to his story, leaders learning to lead may start to understand how powerful storytelling can be in connecting with emotions, images, and subsequent actions. Watch the video now, then answer the following questions.

What are some of the characteristics of Dr. Nordstrom's communication that made his story so compelling?

_____

_____

In what ways did his story connect with you (eg, images and emotions)?

_____

_____

Stephen Denning, in his book, *The Secret Language of Leadership*,[2] describes a model for effective storytelling that includes 3 steps as well as 6 enablers for these steps as portrayed in Figure 5-3. The 3 steps include get attention, stimulate desire, and reinforce messages with reason. Denning elaborates that by continuing the conversation, individuals have the chance to explore, discuss, and gain greater understanding through shared learning. The 6 elements or enablers that help to support or facilitate better storytelling include deploying body language, telling authentically truthful stories, using narrative intelligence, understanding the audience's story, committing to the idea for change (ie, leader's own story), and articulating a clear, inspiring idea for change.

Another model for effective storytelling identifies tips for leaders to convert a good story into a better one.[10] According to this model's guidance, verbal narratives should not be longer than 3 to 5 minutes.[10] Brevity is key to getting the message across to potential followers effectively and efficiently. While ensuring all of the steps for effective storytelling may not be difficult, doing so with brevity takes practice.

A-HA! – STORYTELLING IS A SKILL THAT CAN BE DEVELOPED

Storytelling can be a powerful tool for effectiveness as a leader. While some may find the skill of authentic storytelling comes naturally, many do not. Regardless, this is yet another skill that can be learned, and the models described previously can be put into practice toward mastering your stories.

Consider the models and tips for storytelling. What area(s) do you feel you could use the most work in improving your storytelling?

_____

_____

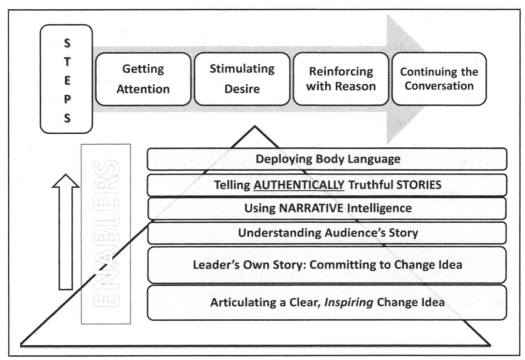

Figure 5-3. A model for effective storytelling. (Reprinted with permission from Denning S. *The Secret Language of Leadership*. San Francisco, CA: John Wiley & Sons, Inc; 2007.)

The Art of Persuasion

A well-told story allows others to see things from your perspective, and, therefore, they are more likely to be influenced and persuaded to follow your ideas and understand your side of the story. Leadership is about influence, and persuasion is a fundamental skill that can directly impact a leader's ability to influence others.

Persuasion involves being able to convince others to take appropriate action. To succeed at engaging others in working toward a common goal or a shared vision, leaders need to answer why people should do something different. Persuasion may be needed to answer this "why" question effectively.[11,12] However, persuasion may be misunderstood as devious tactics, manipulation, or coercion. Without a doubt, persuasion involves moving people to a position they may not currently hold, but persuasion does not need to be done by pleading, coaxing, or threatening. When persuasion is used constructively and assertively, then it becomes a definite learning experience through which the person who is persuading may lead others to fulfilling a shared opportunity or solution.[11]

According to Conger, effective persuasion involves the following 4 distinct and essential steps[11]:
1. Establish credibility.
2. Frame goals and arguments in ways that identify and highlight the collective and common ground.
3. Reinforce desired positions using vivid language and compelling evidence.
4. Connect emotionally with the audience.

When working on the skill of persuasion, leaders should anticipate that the process will take time, energy, and patience. It may be rare to arrive at a shared understanding or a shared solution on the first or even second try. As you learn to be more effective at persuasion, it might be helpful to practice remembering the names of everyone involved in the conversation because it demonstrates that you care about them as individuals, and you care about what they have to say. While learning to lead, avoid using language that seems hesitant, such as "isn't it," "you know," "just," "um mm," and "I mean," because this language may detract from the credibility of your opinion. Instead, leaders should use positive language. For example, instead of saying, "But you are wrong about this," practice saying, "That's a good point, and have you considered this." If possible, compliment the other person. For example, you could tell others that you are impressed with the work they completed in preparation for the conversation or meeting.

Activity 5-7: Storytelling for Persuasion

Think about an authentic story you could tell (or that you have told) that would persuade others to see a situation in a different way or that would motivate them to some action. Think about what you would need to do to communicate your story so that it comes across as sincere, compelling, and inspiring. Write it down. Read it out loud.

_____

_____

_____

_____

_____

_____

_____

_____

_____

_____

_____

_____

Mastering Written and Technological Strategies in Communication

Leaders can increase their effectiveness at communicating if and when they choose the right channels of communication. When writing, leaders need to practice using precise language so that others are not left trying to interpret what message their leaders meant to convey. For example, if instructions need to be put in writing, or if multiple parts or steps need to be communicated, then written communication might be the most appropriate channel. Always consider and choose your words carefully because anything you commit to in writing, on paper or electronically, should be considered a permanent record. Invest time and energy in proofreading everything you write before you distribute it.

Just like verbal and nonverbal communication, written communication involves strategies or approaches. It is important to consider the purpose of your communication and your intended audience. For example, if you are writing a professional letter, use and keep a professional, neutral tone, and make sure the points covered are clear. Alternatively, depending on the relationship or the purpose of the communication, a handwritten note or card may effectively convey a more genuine and personal message. Sometimes, to avoid potentially unpleasant and direct interactions, leaders may choose to use written communication to avoid the discomfort of dealing with people face-to-face. While written communication may often be effective, leaders should not use it to avoid any crucial or potentially emotionally charged conversations. In general, it may be wiser to combine verbal and written communication. Leaders may want to use verbal communication first if issues may be more emotional, and then use written communication as a back-up strategy.

Increasingly, leaders are using technology as an essential mode of communication. This may involve a wide range of adapted face-to-face conversations (eg, Facetime [Apple Inc], video Skype [Skype Communications], and Zoom meetings [Zoom Video Communications]) and written communication through email, text messages, tweets, or simply emojis. Certainly, when used intentionally and strategically, computer-mediated communication may help leaders develop broader relationships.

For example, email can be a practical way to send a message to someone who tends to be hard to reach by telephone, does not work in the same location, or is not located in the same part of country or world (ie, in different time zones). Email is also useful when the information is not time-sensitive; when there is a need to distribute information to many people quickly; when the topic is to review content, an agenda, or directions efficiently prior to a meeting or deadline; or when responding to a memo. It is also strategic to use email as a way to save communication as a reference. However, email is not effective when information is highly confidential, is long and complicated, requires face-to-face discussion, or is emotionally charged so the tone of the message could be misconstrued. When communicating by electronic means, miscommunication occurs frequently, sometimes just because the communication never reaches its intended audience. It is also critical to understand that electronic communication is never private and that any message could be forwarded to other people with or without their knowledge at any time.

A-HA! – ELECTRONIC COMMUNICATION

Think about an electronic message you received from someone and how the message surprised, shocked, or made you angry once you started reading it.

How did you respond to this communication?

_____

_____

If you responded by sending another electronic communication, how did the original sender respond to your response?

_____

_____

How did this communication exchange enhance or interfere with your relationship?

_____

_____

Next, think about a time when you crafted an electronic communication and pushed send, only to realize that you wished you hadn't.

What and how did you convey your message?

_____

_____

Was there a better way to communicate, and if so, how? Why would this have made a difference?

_____

_____

Tips for improving communication effectiveness in both written and technological formats include being concise, stating the intention of the correspondence up front, running grammar and spell checks, having another person read the message prior to sending, holding the message as a draft to reread it before sending, and determining whether a message even needed to be sent. The key is to be intentional and strategic in the method of communication chosen.

Bottom Line!

"The way we communicate with others and with ourselves ultimately determines the quality of our lives." – Tony Robbins, American author, entrepreneur, philanthropist, and life coach

Case Study: Communication or Miscommunication?

Two colleagues work in the same department and have noticeably different styles of interpersonal communication. Both physical therapists have worked in this department approximately 5 years and are equally competent and skilled in patient/client management. In general, both physical therapists can role model the behaviors of effective personal leadership, and both could be ideal candidates to assume the department director position should it become vacant. A normal day yields the typical annoyances when working in a busy, dynamic department, including patient no-shows and cancellations, scheduling changes, ongoing policy and payment changes, late arrivals, new patient evaluations, sick and vacation days, and so on. Therapist A is extremely neat and orderly, maintains a steady schedule, and can be described as having a conservative communication style. Therapist B has an extremely professional, empathetic interpersonal communication style yielding strong connections with her patients/clients and their families, but she often runs over her scheduled appointment times, and she has a busy schedule as well. Both therapists rarely have no-shows or cancellations, although occasionally their patients arrive late.

Change is continuous, the department is growing rapidly, and the typical annoyances are mounting. Therapist A decides to email Therapist B asking if she could pay better attention to managing her patient schedule because her style is perceived to be impacting the productivity of the team in a negative and stressful way. At the end of a long and very busy day, Therapist B reads Therapist A's email.

From this case description, compare the following 2 scenarios and try to anticipate possible outcomes for each:

1. Scenario 1: At the end of a long, busy day, Therapist B opens the email and immediately sends an angry email response. The next day, Therapist A reads Therapist B's response and immediately sends an angry response. Both physical therapists work side-by-side throughout the day without acknowledging their email exchanges at all.

2. Scenario 2: At the end of a long, busy day, Therapist B opens the email sent by Therapist A and decides to "sleep on it" before responding. Over the next couple of days, Therapist B looks for an opportunity to approach Therapist A so that she can acknowledge receipt of the email in person, acknowledge that Therapist A has some feedback for her, and then request a follow-up time to have a conversation over a cup of coffee or lunch.

Unfortunately, Scenario 1 plays itself out too often! In this scenario, communication is spiraling out of control and the relationship is being impacted directly. Real damage is occurring. Behaviors are reactive. Someone (most likely Therapist B) needs to stop the email exchange and the back-and-forth responses or attacks, change the approach to communication, and (hopefully) start to rebuild the relationship through some honest self-reflection, peer feedback, and apologies from both sides.

Scenario 2 depicts the recommended way to approach or respond to Therapist A's initial email. Therapist B makes a conscious decision not to respond, and by doing so, she changes the pattern of communication from reactive to proactive, and prevents the destructive spiral of back-and-forth email responses or attacks. In this way, she may be able to keep the relationship in a holding pattern until she can address it through dialogue. Also, acknowledging the email in a face-to-face manner holds Therapist A accountable for sending the email in the first place. Acknowledging Therapist A's feedback demonstrates responsible, interdependent teamwork. Finally, Therapist B's decision to request a face-to-face meeting—to openly discuss receiving such an email, how the feedback was perceived in terms of tone and choice of words, how it made Therapist B feel, and how Therapist A and Therapist B could work better together (based on the feedback)—may be the most constructive and professional way to model leadership in this scenario.

CHAPTER KEY WORDS

Communication, Storytelling, Persuasion

REFERENCES

1. Shannon CE, Weaver W. *The Mathematical Theory of Communication*. Urbana, IL: University of Illinois Press; 1999.

2. Denning S. *The Secret Language of Leadership: How Leaders Inspire Action Through Narrative*. 1st ed. San Francisco, CA: Jossey-Bass; 2007.

3. Youker R. Using the communications styles instrument for teambuilding. *Proj Manag World J*. 2013;II(VII). https://pmworldjournal.com. Accessed October 7, 2018.

4. Price D. *Well Said! Presentations and Conversations That Get Results*. New York, NY: AMACOM, American Management Association; 2012.

5. Wood P. *SNAP: Making the Most of First Impressions, Body Language, and Charisma*. Novato, CA: New World Library; 2012.

6. Covey SR. *The 7 Habits of Highly Effective People: Restoring the Character Ethic*. First Fireside edition. New York, NY: Fireside Book; 1990.

7. Maxwell JC. *Everyone Communicates, Few Connect: What the Most Effective People Do Differently*. Nashville, TN: Thomas Nelson; 2010.

8. Types of Listening. *Changing Minds*. changingminds.org/techniques/listening/types_listening.htm. Accessed October 23, 2018.

9. TRACOM Group. *Social Style Model*. https://www.tracomcorp.com/social-style-training/model. Accessed October 7, 2018.

10. Smith P. *Lead with a Story: A Guide to Crafting Business Narratives That Captivate, Convince, and Inspire*. New York, NY: AMACOM, American Management Association; 2012.

11. Conger JA. The necessary art of persuasion. *Harv Bus Rev*. 1998;76:84–97.

12. Sinek S. *Start With Why: How Great Leaders Inspire Everyone to Take Action*. London, UK: Penguin; 2009.

Suggested Readings

Denning S. *The Secret Language of Leadership*. San Francisco, CA: John Wiley & Sons, Inc.; 2007.
Mueller K. *Communication From the Inside Out*. Philadelphia, PA: F. A. Davis.; 2010.

Teamwork and Collaboration
Sharing a Vision to Engage, Empower, and Energize Teams

Jennifer Green-Wilson, PT, MBA, EdD
Stacey Zeigler, PT, DPT, MS

As difficult as it is to build a cohesive team, it is not complicated.
— *Patrick Lencioni, American author of* The Five Dysfunctions of a Team

CHAPTER OBJECTIVES

▸ Discuss the need for teamwork in health care.
▸ Define *vision*.
▸ Examine how creating a shared vision enhances teamwork.
▸ Describe how teams develop.
▸ Examine the key characteristics of effective teamwork.
▸ Examine the characteristics of collaboration.
▸ Discuss how leadership skills can optimize team performance.
▸ Self-assess your level of engagement as a team member or team leader.

Green-Wilson J, Zeigler S, eds.
Learning to Lead in Physical Therapy (pp 93-114).
© 2020 Taylor & Francis Group.

Leadership Vignette

Karen M. Hughes, PT, MS, LSS BB

I consider the most effective team experience to be when a diverse group of people who have very different backgrounds, experiences, job responsibilities, and communication styles come together and demonstrate respect for each other, and when each person on this team is truly committed to the common good or to a common purpose. Respect is a fundamental attribute for effective teamwork because it allows for open conversation and dialogue. Diverse opinions need to be shared, heard, listened to, and valued at all times. Respect allows for better collaboration because it creates an environment that is comfortable and safe. When it is safe, then team members become more engaged because they are able to focus on the common good for the team's benefit and do not have to worry about power, position, or who may be thinking what. Also, in these situations, passive-aggressive behaviors are minimized because team members know that they can share their honest opinion, even if it is different from the majority viewpoint, without repercussion.

I consider the most ineffective team experience to be under 2 situations. First is when no common goal, vision, or purpose is set for the team. Team members are unclear about why they need to work together and where the team is going. This creates an impossibility in decision making. Secondly, teams are most ineffective when hierarchy or status exists within the team membership. It is extremely hard for a team to function when the vision is lacking and when the team playing field is not level. In other words, when real or perceived hierarchy exists among team members, then honest and open dialogue becomes guarded. It is important for team members to check their badges at the door; to leave their formal titles, power, and authority outside the team meeting. In this way, everyone can become an integral, equally valued member on the team. Lastly, when team members do not respect each other and the team leader either explicitly or passively allows derogatory comments or personal attacks, then individuals may become disengaged and will avoid sharing honest opinions—especially opinions that may seem controversial—and will lose their focus and commitment to the common good.

I have witnessed the direct impact that hierarchy or an uneven playing field has on team dynamics and how power, formal authority, and position can stifle team performance. For example, at the end of a meeting, team members have told me directly, "I would never have said that if person 'X' had been in the room". In health care, some inherent hierarchy can exist. When team members such as medical directors, certain physicians, or the CEO are absent from team meetings, dialogue can be more open because team members may feel more equal. They will speak openly and honestly and say what they would not say otherwise because they are no longer afraid or influenced by others. This behavior inhibits a team from getting to the root problem of an issue and, hence, you will not determine the best solution or outcome from this team.

The role of the team leader is crucial for team function. I see the team leader with 2 paramount roles. First is to facilitate the team and keep its members focused on the purpose, decision making, and time lines. Second is to create the safe environment and to make sure team members understand that they have a significant role to play and a personal responsibility in the decision-making process and outcome. One way to level the playing field in a health care environment is to call all team members by their first names and not by their titles. This tactic allows all members to realize they are equal partners working on the common vision.

The right people need to be on the right team at the right time to ensure dynamic, collaborative teamwork and high performance. Teams need to be built in a way to ensure diversity of thought, position, experience, and role. The team member selection process needs to be performed carefully, with a clear understanding of the vision and purpose of the team. When working on process improvement projects related to patient care, sometimes managers or supervisors feel they are the best representatives from their areas because they think they know the root issues. However, I would prefer to have the frontline people instead, because they deal with the direct patient care and understand the process more clearly. I often use a process mapping tool to determine if all of the process owners are represented. We need to identify who we are missing, and then I recruit them.

THE NEED FOR TEAMWORK AND COLLABORATION

Developing the ability to lead others and to work in teams cooperatively is emphasized as a top priority for leadership development in health care,[1] since poor performance in these areas has been linked to the majority of health care errors.[2,3] Just as much as the development of overt clinical skills, the intentional development of non-technical skills such as leadership, teamwork, management, and communication is needed to help improve patient safety.[4]

As a future or current health care professional, you must understand how to be engaged as a valuable member on any team, and how to fuel and refuel collaborative and dynamic teamwork to ensure patient safety and quality outcomes and transform or advance clinical practice. In this chapter, the skills needed to lead others productively and to enhance teamwork while in leadership roles (eg, team leader and team member) will be examined. Ultimately, the goal is to ignite inclusive teams that are collaborative, high-performing, and ready to embrace change.

SHARING A VISION

In every chapter of this book thus far, "vision" has been mentioned because those who lead have a vision. A *vision* is something you imagine or hope could be in the future. Particularly in Chapter 2, inspiring a shared vision was noted as one of the 5 practices of the exemplary leader, as identified by Kouzes and Posner.[5] Now that the discussion has shifted to leading others, the concept of a vision is particularly important as it is the tie that binds the effective group together.

A *vision statement* can be seen as an ambitious description of an ideal and unique image of the future; it is what a team would like to achieve or accomplish, and it is intended to guide current and future courses of action. Examples of vision statements are listed in Box 6-1.

A great vision is more than just words, however. A great vision is a shared vision among the people attempting to fulfill it. A shared vision helps align, connect, and engage all team members because, through crafting the vision together, team members become united in common values and goals, creating a culture of responsibility. The shared vision encourages the well-coordinated and collaborative actions[6] needed in health care, and each member of an effective team leads toward this vision.

A-HA! – YOUR PART IN THE VISION

Whether you were on the team that helped create the vision, or whether you are part of the team to help reach the already established vision, the vision's existence helps ensure that the team has a clearly defined goal and common purpose to keep the team focused and its work prioritized.[7]

Box 6-1

EXAMPLES OF VISION STATEMENTS

Vision Statement for the Physical Therapy Profession (American Physical Therapy Association)
Transforming society by optimizing movement to improve the human experience.
[Available at: http://www.apta.org/vision/. Accessed: September 9, 2018]

Vision Statement for Habitat for Humanity
A world where everyone has a decent place to live.
[Available at: https://www.hfhsloco.org/about/history-of-habitat-for-humanity/. Accessed: September 9, 2018]

Vision Statement for the American Society for the Prevention of Cruelty to Animals
That the United States is a humane community in which all animals are treated with respect and kindness.
Available at: https://www.aspca.org/about-us/aspca-policy-and-position-statements/vision. Accessed: September 9, 2018

Which of the visions listed in Box 6-1 resonates with you the most, and why?

_____

_____

_____

The last time you were part of a team, did the group create a shared vision, or was it working toward an already existing vision?

_____

_____

_____

Were all team members clear on what the vision for the group was? How did this affect the function of the group?

_____

_____

_____

What was your role in creating or fulfilling the vision?

_____

_____

_____

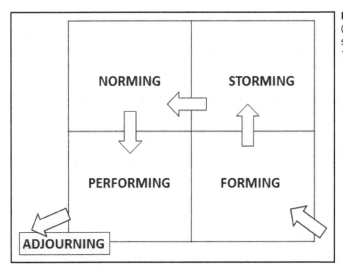

Figure 6-1. Stages of team development. (Adapted from Tuckman B. Developmental sequence in small groups. *Psychol Bull.* 1965;63[6]:384-399.)

> **Bottom Line!**
>
> Leaders have a vision. Those who follow share that vision and may have even helped to create that vision. Those who lead include everyone on the team working toward the shared vision. The vision becomes a reality when everyone leads effectively at all levels.

HOW TEAMS FORM AND TRANSFORM

Teams are groups of people who share a common purpose, work together to achieve specific goals, and are mutually committed to these goals and to each other. This contrasts with *groups*, which simply develop when a collection of individuals coordinates its individual efforts in various ways. Groups and group dynamics are not dependent on being a team, but teams do need good group dynamics.

Stages of Team Development

The Tuckman model, a well-known approach used to understand group or team development, identifies 5 progressive stages of formation: forming, storming, norming, performing, and adjourning (Figure 6-1).[8]

This model provides valuable insight because it emphasizes that relationships can become established within teams, and team leaders can be more effective when they change or adapt their leadership styles as the teams develop in maturity, interdependence, accountability, and ability.

While forming (stage 1), the team has a high dependence on the leader for guidance and direction; individual roles and responsibilities are unclear; processes are often ignored or under-developed; and the team leader must be prepared to answer many questions about the team's purpose, objectives, and external relationships. In this stage, the leader tends to use a directing or telling style of leadership.

During the storming stage (stage 2), decisions are not made easily; cliques and subgroups form; power struggles may emerge as team members attempt to establish themselves in relation to other team members; and the leader may become challenged by certain team members. Even though the team has a clearer sense of purpose, many uncertainties may still exist. The leader needs to use a coaching style to keep the team focused on its goals and to avoid becoming distracted by relationships and emotional issues. Ultimately, at this stage, compromises may be needed to enable progress.

By the norming stage (stage 3), agreement and consensus form, roles and responsibilities are clear and generally accepted, critical decisions are made, and members can openly discuss and develop processes and working style. Moreover, the team generally respects the leader, commitment and unity are strong, and the team shares some of the leadership. The leader can succeed by using a participative style to facilitate and enable the completion of the required work.

By the performing stage (stage 4), the team knows clearly why it is doing what it is doing, it works productively toward achieving its goals, and it pays attention to relationships and process issues. The team has developed a high degree of autonomy, and even though disagreements may still occur, these may be successfully resolved. The leader is comfortable with empowering or delegating to other team members because the team now has its own capacity to make most of its own decisions, relying on previously agreed upon ground rules and criteria.

The final stage of team development (stage 5) is when the team adjourns. While this may not seem like a developmental stage, it is worthy of recognition because the team members who like routine or who have developed close relationships with their team members could find this stage to be the most difficult of all. Team leaders are wise to recognize and help prepare the group for its ultimate disbandment possibly through a review of the team's work, acknowledgment of the team's process and performance, and the value of the relationships that made the group flourish.

A-HA! – YOUR LAST TEAM

Think of the last team that you were on, and ask yourself the following questions:
Was it an effective team? Why or why not?

_____

_____

_____

Based on the stages of team development in Figure 6-1, did your team appear to go through each stage naturally, or did it get stuck at any point?

_____

_____

_____

How did the flow of the stages appear to affect the team's effectiveness? Linear fashion, or back-and-forth?

_____

_____

_____

Types of Teams

Performance is influenced by the way in which and the reasons why teams are structured in certain ways. In other words, a correlation may exist between team structure and the team's ability to produce. The curve found in Johnson and Johnson's book, _Joining Together: Group Theory & Group Skills_, identifies the following 4 types of teams[9]:

1. Pseudogroups
2. Traditional groups or teams
3. Effective teams
4. High-performance teams

A *pseudogroup* is a group whose members have been assigned to work together but do not have any real interest in doing so. Even though team members talk to each other, they may actually view each other as rivals and, therefore, may compete with one another. As a result, they may not trust each other fully, may withhold information, may attempt to mislead and confuse, or may even block performance intentionally or unintentionally.

A *traditional team* is a group whose members accept that they have to work together, but may still see little long-term benefit from doing so. This structure promotes individualistic work with members being most productive when working alone. Generally, the team does not develop because members have minimal to no interest in or commitment to one another or to the team's collective success or output. An example of this type of team would be the formation of a student group selected by faculty, in which some students contribute, prepare, and conduct research for the upcoming team presentation, while others contribute little or nothing.

In contrast, an *effective team* is one in which its members work together to accomplish shared goals. Members perceive that they can reach their goals if and only if the other team members also reach their goals. An example of this type of team would be if a student group decided to divide and conquer the collective work needed to be completed, and then each member delivered individual assignments on time and done well. Next, this team worked together cooperatively to organize and seamlessly integrate the pieces for a team presentation.

Finally, a *high-performance team* can be distinguished from an effective one by the level of commitment members have to one another and to the team's success. These teams typically outperform all acceptable expectations, given their membership. Engaged and committed high-performing teams can achieve transformational outcomes.

A noteworthy example of a consistently high-performing team is a self-directed team, with individuals from various entities who collaborate on a specific project or task. These individuals bring their expertise to develop a program, design or redesign a process, or initiate a new strategy. Besides coming together to achieve a common goal, successful self-directed teams require other conditions or characteristics including joint responsibility, interdependence, and empowerment.[10] Self-directed teams assign responsibility to all members of the group. This joint responsibility creates a sense of ownership for each team member and allows each member to feel fully invested in their collective success.[10] As team members feel more fully invested, they may work harder to see their team succeed. Moreover, the sense of interdependence among team members increases the success of self-directed teams.

A-HA! – YOUR LAST TEAM (REVISITED)

Using the same team experience you described in A-Ha! – Your Last Team on page 98, decide which kind of team it was from the descriptions in this section.

Was your team a pseudogroup, traditional team, effective team, or high-performing team?

_____

What did the team members and/or team leader(s) do to make this experience what it was?

_____

_____

_____

TABLE 6-1. PERSONAL ROLE IN TEAM: SELF-ASSESSMENT

Directions: As you may behave differently depending on the situation, self-assess each item below based on how you feel _most typically_ in a team.

	NEVER	SOMETIMES	ALWAYS
I try to include other members in group activities.			
I am influenced by other group members.			
I discuss my ideas, feelings, and reactions to what is taking place within the group.			
I express acceptance and support when other members disclose their ideas, feelings, and reactions to what is taking place in the group.			

Adapted from Johnson DW, Johnson FP. *Joining Together: Group Theory & Group Skills.* 10th ed. Upper Saddle River, NJ: Pearson; 2009.

How would you describe the role that you played in this team's function?

_____

_____

_____

Activity 6-1: Your Impact on the Team Self-Assessment

Teams are a set of interpersonal relationships structured and fueled by a compelling, distinct, and specific purpose that requires the joint efforts as well as individual tangible contributions.[9] Now that you have reflected upon your last team experience, take a few moments to assess how your behaviors can impact the cohesiveness of your team (Table 6-1).[9] What can you summarize about the impact you have on a team?

The Role of the Team Leader

A *team leader's* role is to inspire a vision that others can contribute to and share. By listening and talking to team members about hopes, dreams, and passions, leaders can start to discern what is meaningful to others, find common ground, and give a collective voice to members' feelings, passions, and aspirations. A leader can be effective in the long run when time is spent helping others understand how their individual needs can be satisfied in addition to the team's shared goals.[5]

In general, the most productive and innovative teams are led by team leaders who are both task-oriented and relationship-oriented, and who are able to adapt their styles over time and based on the team's needs.[11] Ideally, what may work the best is when team leaders are more task-focused at the beginning of team formation, and then are able to shift toward more of a relationship-oriented approach once the team's work is well underway.[11] Recall in Chapter 2, Kouzes and Posner proposed "model the way" as one of the 5 practices of exemplary leaders.[5] Leaders set the example by demonstrating or modeling behaviors they expect of others. Team leaders should role-model explicitly the expected and desired collaborative behaviors for the rest of the team. In this way, team leaders set the tone and expectation for what collaboration looks like.

Recall also in Chapter 2 that exemplary team leaders believe passionately they can make a difference, and, therefore, they model passion by being enthusiastic when they interact with others.[5] Effective team leaders create time to envision the future, listen closely for shared goals, and recruit and engage others to examine forward-looking opportunities together.[5] Exemplary team leaders challenge the process and their teams, search for opportunities to change the status quo, and look for innovative ways to improve the organization or group through risk-taking and experimentation.[5] Exemplary team leaders strengthen entire teams by increasing self-determination and self-motivation in others, and by developing competence. Finally, exemplary team leaders know the value to be gained by sincerely recognizing and celebrating the contributions made by each team member, as well as acknowledging the many small wins and positive steps achieved throughout the team process. In this way, team members feel valued and appreciated and, therefore, stay actively engaged in moving forward collectively.[5]

Bottom Line!

An effective team process is not just about the what, or the outcome. Effective teams figure out *how* they want to work together to succeed in working toward the shared vision.

COLLABORATIVE TEAMS

According to the Cambridge English Dictionary,[12] *collaboration* is defined as "the situation of 2 or more people working together to create or achieve the same thing." Creating a collaborative team environment is essential for teams to succeed.[7] In fact, creating the right team environment and the right conditions for teamwork accounts for approximately 60% of the variation in how well a team eventually performs, while the quality of how a team is launched accounts for another 30%.[13] Therefore, collaboration can be directly impacted when team leaders and team members invest in creating the right conditions and in launching their teams well from the very beginning.[13] Ideally, all team members have a responsibility to lead themselves and others depending on the situation and the needs of the team. All of the leadership skills mentioned thus far can be used to do this.

Collaborative Team Composition

It is important to be selective as to how many people should be on the team, as well as who needs to be recruited, with a focus on the skills, knowledge, and experiences needed to form a well-rounded team for each particular assignment. Ideally, each team wants its members to be willing and capable of forming a cohesive group because cohesiveness is often linked to the team's productivity level. Some may decide to form teams with homogeneous skills, experiences, and styles because it may seem easier to build this cohesiveness when its team members seem similar or like-minded. However, these homogeneous teams may be missing some diverse perspectives, skills, or experiences needed to yield different or more creative results. Therefore, team members need to work at seeking, welcoming, and embracing new ideas and fresh perspectives, and not ignoring them or pushing them aside.

Cooperation increases when the roles of individual team members are clarified and defined clearly, and when the team is given latitude on how to achieve its task.[11] Knowing everyone's role and being familiar with the responsibility of those roles will create efficiency and flexibility in how the team completes its work. Measuring and monitoring team output as well as the team's internal group dynamics and relationships may provide valuable information so that the team does not become derailed. In other words, it may be helpful for collaborative teams to assign a few team members to monitor task needs and a few others to monitor relationship needs, and then regularly review and evaluate the effectiveness of team meetings to make sure the team process is still meeting everyone's needs.[7]

Edward de Bono, in his book, *Six Thinking Hats*,[14] describes a simple yet effective parallel or lateral thinking process that can help teams be more focused, creative, and thoughtfully engaged. It can

TABLE 6-2. THINKING DIFFERENTLY: SIX HATS OR SIX ROLES

HAT COLOR	DESCRIPTION
Blue	Manage the process (facilitator role) Next steps, decisions made, action plans
Red	Feelings, hunches, perceptions, instinct, and intuition
Yellow	Values and benefits, why something may work, optimistic
Black	Difficulties, potential problems, why something may not work, pessimistic
Green	Creativity, solutions, alternatives, new ideas (eg, brainstorming)
White	Data, facts, information known or needed

Reprinted with permission from DeBono E. *Six Thinking Hats*. New York, NY: Little Brown and Company; 1999.

be used to facilitate a more effective (and possibly more efficient) group decision-making process. When using this model, each person learns how to separate thinking into 6 well-defined functions and roles. Each thinking role is identified with a colored, symbolic "thinking hat." For example, the Red Hat is used to get team members to express emotions and feelings and share fears, likes, dislikes, loves, and hates, whereas, the Green Hat is focused on creativity, possibilities, alternatives, and new ideas. By mentally wearing and switching hats, team members can focus or redirect ideas, the conversation, or the meeting itself. Everyone must use the same hat at the same time to ensure parallel thinking rather than argument. The hats are not about personal preference or personality types; rather, they are used to encourage each member of the group to contribute to all aspects of the thinking (Table 6-2[14]).

Also noteworthy in discussing collaborative team composition is that individuals tend to act differently when they are in teams as compared to how they behave as individuals. Behaviors of formal teams are shaped by the common purpose and shared goals, whereas informal groups seem more like alliances that may or may not be guided by formality depending on the groups' interests and need for social interaction and engagement. Team members interact by exchanging verbal, nonverbal, and written messages that influence each other. As such, team leaders and team members who want to be effective at influencing team behavior must understand that a team's behavior is influenced both by the individuals within the team as well as the dynamics of the collective group of individuals. Learning about the professional and personal roles of each member of the team at the start of a team experience can provide some insight into possible patterns of individual and team behavior. Taking time to learn about the motivations for each team member will also be valuable to keep the team energized. Team leaders and team members can shape, define, and model the desirable behaviors proactively for the team and, ultimately, influence standards for effective team group behavior.[9]

A-HA! – YOU IN DIFFERENT CONTEXTS

Do you tend to behave the same or do you behave differently when you are on a team as compared to how you behave when you work as an individual?

_____

_____

TABLE 6-3. EFFECTIVE VERSUS INEFFECTIVE TEAMS		
DIMENSION	**EFFECTIVE TEAMS**	**INEFFECTIVE TEAMS**
Goals	Goals are continually clarified and modified to reflect and include ideas, needs, and feelings of all team members; build buy-in and commitment from all team members; and attempt to align individual goals with team goals.	Goals are imposed, assigned, and enforced. Team members may tend to compete against each other.
Communication	Characterized by an ongoing dialogue that is 2-way and open to allow honest sharing of feelings and ideas.	Characterized by a monologue or 1-way communication. Feelings may be suppressed or ignored.
Participation	All team members are actively engaged. How the team members work together transforms over time and with experience.	Participation is unequal, and high-power members dominate. Some social loafing occurs within team, with a person exerting less effort to achieve a goal when working in a group than when working alone. The focus is on the task, not the people or relationships.
Leadership	Responsibility and accountability for the team's leadership are shared.	Leadership of the team is in the hands of a few individuals, sometimes based on ability. Tasks are often dictated or assigned.
Power and influence	Power is equalized and shared to ensure that individuals' goals and needs are fulfilled, and all abilities are used and valued.	The role within the team determines power. Conformity to the team leader is expected (ie, team members need to do what they have been told to do).

(continued)

Try to identify specific behaviors that may be the same or different. Why do you think you behave differently in these situations?

_____

_____

Collaborative Team Environment

Productive teams need to invest energy and time upfront to develop strategies aimed at enhancing cohesiveness, minimizing team insulation, and establishing ground rules and procedures that will

TABLE 6-3 (CONTINUED). EFFECTIVE VERSUS INEFFECTIVE TEAMS

DIMENSION	EFFECTIVE TEAMS	INEFFECTIVE TEAMS
Decision making	Team members decide proactively how they want to make decisions, and methods may be used at different times to match the needs of the situation. Involvement and group discussions are encouraged, and critical decisions may be made by consensus, if possible.	The team leader or a select few make decisions. Team member involvement and discussions are minimal. Quick compromises are made to eliminate any arguing. Groupthink may be prevalent.
Conflict	Different opinions are allowed so that all team members can advocate openly for their own views and challenge each other's assumptions and opinions. Conflict is seen as vital for achieving high-quality, creative decision making and problem solving.	Conflicts are resolved using a win-lose approach, avoided, or ignored.
Team function	Characterized by inclusion, friendliness, respect, acceptance, encouragement, and trust. Allows the team to develop and become more cohesive over time and with experience.	Individual work is the norm. Rigid conformity is endorsed. Group cohesion is ignored.

Reprinted with permission from Johnson DW, Johnson FP. *Joining Together: Group Theory & Group Skills.* 10th ed. Upper Saddle River, NJ: Pearson; 2009.

allow diverse options to be discussed and ensure consensus-driven decision making.[15] Both team members and the designated team leader play key roles in ensuring that each person on the team has a voice and feels valued. Essentially, an effective or productive team will be measured not only by whether it achieves its goals, but also by how well it maintains valuable working relationships among its members and adapts to changing conditions or needs within and outside of the team. When team leaders and team members take time proactively to understand characteristics of effective and ineffective groups, then they can focus more clearly on how they can lead their team and how they can transform any ineffective team behaviors to become more effective and productive.

Johnson and Johnson, in their book, *Joining Together: Group Theory & Group Skills*, detail both effective and ineffective team function (Table 6-3).[9]

Johnson and Johnson have also identified guidelines to provide direction for creating effective teams and a framework for analyzing how well the teams are functioning. These guidelines are straightforward and useful for leaders learning to lead, and are summarized in Box 6-2.[9]

A-HA! – EFFECTIVE AND INEFFECTIVE TEAMS

Review the characteristics of effective teams as listed in Table 6-3 and the guidelines for creating effective teams in Box 6-2. Reflect on a few of your team experiences to answer the following questions:

How many of the guidelines in Box 6-2 did your team follow?

Box 6-2

GUIDELINES FOR CREATING EFFECTIVE TEAMS

- Establish relevant, well-defined team goals that include a high level of commitment and accountability from every team member.
- Establish productive 2-way communication so that all team members feel included and encouraged to openly and accurately communicate their ideas, opinions, and feelings.
- Encourage and ensure that all team members participate.
- Ensure that leadership is shared and adapted to meet the needs of the team. Ensure the use of power is distributed among team members.
- Decide how decisions will be made as a team based on the time and resources available, the magnitude and importance of the decisions, and the team member commitment needed to implement them.
- Allow structured disagreements so that team members can advocate their views, disagree, and challenge each other's assumptions; see also Chapter 8 regarding orchestrating conflict.

Adapted from Johnson DW, Johnson FP. *Joining Together: Group Theory & Group Skills.* 10th ed. Upper Saddle River, NJ: Pearson-Prentice Hall; 1999.

If these guidelines were used, how did they help?

_____

If these guidelines were not used, how could they have helped improve the performance of the team? Why?

_____

What else could have been done to improve the dynamics of the team? Why?

_____

●━━━━━━━━━━━━━━━━

Collaborative Team Function

Now that we have considered both team formation and team environment, team function during its longevity may be the most challenging. Team collaboration can be impacted significantly when each team member and the team itself can invest in learning how to build relationships, communicate well, and resolve conflicts creatively.[11] Patrick Lencioni echoes this as he describes the 5 foundational functions (opposite of *dysfunctions*) for effective teamwork, including[16]:

1. Team members trust one another.
2. Team members engage in unfiltered conflict around ideas.
3. Team members commit to decisions and action plans.
4. Team members hold each other and one another accountable for delivering results.
5. Team members focus on achievement of collective results.

Contrary to the 5 foundational functions for effective teamwork are the 5 dysfunctions.[16] The 5 dysfunctions of a team detail patterns of behavior that limit team performance and include absence of trust, fear of conflict, lack of commitment, avoidance of accountability, and inattention to results. In this model, trust is viewed as the most foundational aspect needed for building functional teams.

Activity 6-2: Practice Creating and Sustaining an Effective Team

- Step 1: Read the following scenario:
  - ○ Jenny, Marcia, and Joan decided to work as a team to complete a student group project required for one of their professional issues classes. This project was worth 40% of their final course grade. All 3 of these students preferred to be the team leader. They spent a fair amount of time initially deciding how they wanted to do their work, and then when they should have certain parts of the project completed. After their first team meeting, Jenny left feeling somewhat angry because not only did she feel like she deserved to be the group leader, but she also did not like the project design suggestions made by Marcia and Joan. During the second team meeting, Marcia showed up 15 minutes late, and then Jenny took time trying to persuade Marcia and Joan to see her point regarding how the project should be completed. Joan left this second meeting feeling frustrated. As the deadline quickly approached, Jenny and Joan completed the work that they had been "assigned," while Marcia consistently missed each deadline. Tensions started to build among the team members, and each team member perceived that the work was not being satisfactorily completed.
- Step 2: Team dysfunction: Imagine that you are the team leader dealing with this ineffective team function. Based on Lencioni's 5 dysfunctions,[16] analyze the scenario for aspects that might be dysfunctional at this point.
- Step 3: Individual dysfunction: Consider 4 challenging behaviors commonly found in individuals and whole teams, including passive uninvolvement, active uninvolvement, independence, and taking charge (Table 6-4).[9] Analyze the behaviors of individuals in the scenario and determine a leadership strategy to help turn things around using the Suggested Strategy column in Table 6-4.

One final piece that has not been mentioned that may affect team function is groupthink. *Groupthink* refers to the type of thinking or belief that is often forced upon the entire group. In these situations, agreement and consensus are expected, and any alternative or unpopular views are overruled. Collective pressure is placed on all members to conform, while skeptics or those with minority opinions are persuaded to support the option favored by the vocal majority. Nonbelievers keep silent and minimize their hesitations and doubts to project an appearance of consensus and to avoid rocking the boat. The group then translates this silence as support for or as a "yes" vote for the majority, creating a shared illusion of unanimity (ie, members *always* agree with each other).[17,18] Groups who experience groupthink are more likely to be dogmatic, characterized by opinions being expressed very strongly or positively as if they were facts. Also, members of the in-group (majority) may stereotype members of the out-group (minority) as malicious, uncommitted, or irresponsible, and exclude or marginalize them.[18] Variables to look for, correlated with times when groupthink tends to emerge, include:

- When the team or group is extremely cohesive
- When the leader is directive, opinionated, energetic, and purposeful
- When the team is isolated from outsiders and outside criticism/feedback
- When there are time pressures and clear deadlines to perform
- When the team fails to apply a methodical decision-making process to analytically evaluate alternatives

The cure for groupthink is prevention. By following the successful collaborative team formation, environment, and function tips provided in this section, groupthink can largely be prevented. If it

TABLE 6-4. STRATEGIES FOR DEALING WITH CHALLENGING BEHAVIORS FOUND IN TEAMS		
BEHAVIORAL ISSUE	**EXAMPLE**	**SUGGESTED STRATEGY**
Passively uninvolved	Team members do not participate in or pay attention to the work needed to be done; they say little or nothing during team meetings and show no enthusiasm. They come to meetings unprepared (often late) and without their materials and resources.	If this team member does not contribute information voluntarily, then other team members need to ask directly (in-person, possibly one-on-one) for the information and hold this team member accountable to produce it. Divide up the roles and assign this team member a role that is essential to the success of the team.
Actively uninvolved	Team member talks about everything but the work that needs to be done; refuses to do the work; refuses to work with another team member; and/or shows up late or leaves team meetings early.	Assign this team member a specific role. Make this team member accountable for the coordination and overall functioning of the tasks. Confront this team member if needed; give constructive feedback.
Independent	Team member works alone and, essentially, ignores the team discussion.	Rearrange the work so that this member cannot complete the work without relying on another member for information, thereby forcing collaboration and interaction.
(Too) Assertive (ie, takes charge)	One team member does all the work, refuses to let other members participate, orders members around, or makes decisions for the team without checking to see if other members agree with these decisions.	Assign roles so that other team members have equal or more influential roles on the team. Establish ground rules for how the team will make its decisions. Confront this team member; give constructive feedback.
Adapted from Johnson DW, Johnson FP. *Joining Together: Group Theory & Group Skills.* 10th ed. Upper Saddle River, NJ: Pearson; 2009:551-552.		

occurs despite best efforts, analyze the team for function and dysfunction to implement the effective leadership strategies discussed thus far in this chapter.

Bottom Line!

As a team leader and as a team member, it is important to understand why a team exists, how to structure and form successfully, how to create a collaborative environment, and how to continually assess its function. Then, the collective team will be able to decide how to lead the team most effectively together.

OPTIMIZING TEAM PERFORMANCE

The good news is that team performance can be optimized through intentional thought and action. Building trust, empowering, and engaging team members while using power wisely are stepping-stones to effective teamwork and are the focus of this next section.

Building Trust Amongst Team Members

Trust is the belief that someone is good or honest, or that something is reliable or safe. It is logical, then, that trust is a foundational ingredient for effective teamwork. Lencioni's model identified that team members trust one another in functioning teams, and that when trust is absent, this absence or lack of trust becomes a behavior that limits performance.[16] In imagining a team in which a high level of trust exists, the energy of the group may be palpable; all team members would be open, candid, and authentic in sharing their ideas and opinions; information would be shared with everyone; and the real issues would be confronted.[19] Additionally, in this team, there would be a sincere sense of accountability and commitment, innovation and creativity would be stimulated, individuals may become more tolerant of mistakes, people would share the credit abundantly, and there would be few "meetings after meetings."[19] In contrast, imagine a team in which trust is low or lacking. This team may exhibit the following behaviors: tension may be palpable while the general energy level of the team is low and sluggish; team members may withhold, manipulate, or distort critical information needed for decision making; and team members may openly resist or stifle new ideas. Moreover, team members may tend to overpromise and underdeliver, and, in this case, no one holds each other accountable when deadlines are missed.[19]

Within a team, the level of trust changes continuously, and it depends upon team members being willing and able to be trusting and trustworthy. Interpersonal trust is built when individuals take risks, are vulnerable and self-disclosing, and are openly accepting and supportive of others.[9] Self-disclosure is at the core of relationship development, and when one person is not able or willing to self-disclose information, then it may stop others from self-disclosing as well. Team leaders and team members need to be cooperative, open, and authentic with each other and willing to share or self-disclose their own thoughts, feelings, needs, aspirations, fears, likes, and dislikes to work together effectively as trustworthy team members.

A-HA! – TRUST IN SELF AND TRUST IN OTHERS

In Chapter 2, you assessed your self-trust using the items in Table 2-3. Review your results, and answer the following questions with application to trusting others.

Do you trust yourself?

_____

Are you generally trusting of others?

_____

What does it take for you to trust someone else?

_____

How do your answers relate to the trust you have in others on your team(s)?

_____

Power and Influence When Leading Teams

When asked about the connection between power and leadership, people typically focus on the control and decision-making pressures that leaders can exert in their formal leadership roles. In this way, leaders are seen as powerful because they can make things happen. Others who tend to view the concept of power with discomfort react cautiously when asked to describe the power that leaders have or need to have to be effective in their role. Power gives a leader the capacity or potential to influence, and through influence, leaders can affect and possibly change others' beliefs, attitudes, and actions. Leaders—formal and informal—at all levels have access to some forms of power, yet often, power is either underused or not realized. Because power can translate into control, authority, or influence over others, it is important to understand and be aware of the dynamic association between power and leadership, as well as to understand how to access sources of power to be an effective team leader.

In learning to lead, power is a fundamental concern for leaders and followers and for their relationships.[20] The bases of social power have been identified as legitimate, reward, coercive, expert, and referent, and further categorized as either positional or personal.[20] *Positional power*, associated with formal leadership roles, is derived from rank or responsibility in an organization. Legitimate, reward, and coercive bases of power are associated with this positional type of power. *Legitimate power* is formal power or authority associated with or derived from a formal position or role. *Reward* and *coercive power* can be used by formal leaders if and when they decide to compensate, recognize, and reward followers, or assign consequences to discipline them. In contrast, *personal power* is essentially derived from being seen as likeable, approachable, and knowledgeable and can be leveraged in both formal and informal leadership roles depending on the relationships with others. *Referent* and *expert* are bases of power linked to this personal type of power. Expert power is derived when followers consider their leader to be the expert and competent, thereby giving the leader the power and influence over decisions, situations, and people and teams. For example, when patients/clients (followers) view their physical therapists as experts, then the physical therapists (clinician-leaders) have access to the power or influence they can use to motivate others to make behavioral or lifestyle changes. Alternatively, referent power is given to leaders because the followers like and choose to follow the leader. Then, when followers decide to follow a certain leader, this relationship can be powerful and transformational.

Leaders can strengthen their access to power, especially referent power, when they spend time trying to understand why followers choose to follow someone, or not, as a way to understand leadership more deeply. Recall from Chapters 2 and 3, a leader is only a leader if there are followers (with your first follower being you). The reasons why followers follow can vary, and sometimes they can be complex. For example, some followers follow a leader out of fear, while in other situations, followers perceive some benefit or some value to be gained from the relationship. Followers choose to follow a leader when trust exists in the relationship, when the leader's values and goals align with their own values and goals, and when followers are mutually invested in a shared vision or goal.

Empowering and Engaging Team Members

It is easy to confuse the concepts of delegation and empowerment, and important for those who lead to know the difference. When team leaders *delegate*, they assign tasks to their team members. When a task is delegated, the assigned team member may be expected to follow a certain set of rules or protocol, and may be required to check in frequently with the team leader to make sure the team member remains on-task. In this situation, creativity and initiative may be limited.

Alternatively, when leaders *empower*, they assign ownership, responsibility, and accountability to others, in addition to the task. Empowerment involves encouraging others to own what they do and how they do it; it involves trust and accountability based on a set of knowledge, skills, experiences, and level of motivation. Essentially, empowerment may be described as the practice of sharing

---

Box 6-3

LEVELS OF ENGAGEMENT

- Engaged employees are passionate in their work and feel connected to their team and organization; they drive innovation and move the team/organization forward.
- Passively engaged employees go through the motions of work but lack energy and passion.
- Actively disengaged employees are unhappy at work and tell their coworkers how unhappy they are. They tend to undermine the accomplishments of those who are engaged in their work

Reprinted with permission from State of the American Workplace: Employee Engagement Insights for US Business Leaders. Gallup, Inc.; 2014. Available at: http://www.gallup.com/poll/165269/worldwide-employees-engaged-work.aspx. Accessed September 10, 2018.

---

information and power with team members so that they can take initiative, make decisions to solve problems, and implement solutions. Empowerment is based on the belief that by giving team members opportunity, resources, and authority, as well holding them responsible and accountable for the outcomes of their actions, they will have the necessary means, motivation, and level of satisfaction to perform—and to perform well. Ultimately, empowerment can improve performance.

Empowerment fosters engagement, and there is a strong link between engagement and performance. Engagement has been characterized by vigor, absorption, and dedication, as described here[21-23]:

- *Vigor* refers to people being physically active in their work, even when the work is essentially sedentary or deskbound, and it helps people sustain their effort even when they meet challenges or obstacles. Vigor means that people are physically energized, are mentally strong, and put significant effort into their work.
- *Absorption* refers to when individuals become so engrossed in their work that they lose track of time, surroundings, and other people.
- *Dedication* means that individuals display high levels of enthusiasm and devotion to their work because they find it so meaningful and fulfilling.

An engaged team looks happier and busier, and research has confirmed that engaged workers have higher job satisfaction, work harder, and perform better than their less engaged colleagues.[24] Engaged team members inspire innovation, and passionate teams are most likely to drive organizations forward.[24] Research shows that engagement is strongly connected to outcomes essential for financial success, including productivity, profitability, and customer satisfaction.[24] Engagement may be influenced by an individual's levels of optimism, self-efficacy, and self-esteem, plus the autonomy to do the work and make decisions. Access to coaching and feedback on performance may also impact engagement. Other factors that may influence engagement directly include a presence of trust and integrity, the ability to align individual effort with team performance, a presence of professional growth opportunities, good working relationships with colleagues, and a strong relationship with the immediate or direct (formal) manager or supervisor.[21] Whether a team member is engaged, passively engaged, or actively disengaged (Box 6-3[25]), the result has a large impact on team performance.

Activity 6-3: How Engaged Are You?

Think about the teams in which you are a team member or a team leader—professionally, personally, or academically. Ask yourself the following questions to get an idea about your level of engagement.

Are you passionate about your work? _____

Do you dedicate time and energy to your work? _____

Do you make your work a priority? _____

Do you often get distracted? _____

What kind of team member do you think you are? _____

_____

Review your responses and write a few ideas on how you could increase your level of engagement (even if you perceive yourself as already engaged)?

_____

_____

_____

Keeping Teams Energized

Creating a shared vision inspires and provides focus for team energy. Team members typically expect team leaders to be inspiring and to stimulate this shared and compelling vision— over and over again—but both team leaders and team members need to be stewards or overseers of team energy.[26] This means that teams need to know when to ignite energy and enthusiasm, and when to allow time to refuel.

Of all people working, 74% are experiencing a personal energy crisis.[27] Only 56% of employees feel physically energized at work.[27] People seem to be working more hours; spending more time tied to digital devices and technology; and taking less time to reflect, renew, and prioritize. As a result, people may feel exhausted, overwhelmed, and possibly disengaged. To perform at their best, people require 4 sources of energy: physical, emotional, mental, and spiritual.[26] All sources are necessary for optimal performance; no one source of energy is adequate enough by itself.

Activity 6-4: How Energized Are You?

Take a few moments to examine your energy level, and then reflect upon a few areas where you might need to make some changes with these guided questions. For a quick self-assessment, it may be helpful to take the Johnson & Johnson Human Performance Institute free energy survey available at https://energyprofile.perfprog.com/free.[28]

Is there a potential source of energy you feel more challenged by than others when it comes to your own personal energy? Why?

_____

_____

_____

Identify one behavior that you are not doing currently but know you should, and write a goal for the yourself to make this behavioral change to boost your energy right away.

_____

_____

_____

Those who choose to lead need to model methods for staying fueled, meaning taking time to invest in themselves. Exercising, getting sufficient rest, eating the right types of food, and staying attuned to passions all contribute to good leadership behavior. Investing in relationship building is another way to remain fueled.[29] When individual members of the team practice good leadership, the whole team wins.

A-HA! – DO YOU REFUEL?

Reflect upon how proactive you are at balancing the physical, mental, social/emotional, and spiritual needs and demands in your life.[29]

What are your areas of strength?

_____

_____

_____

What areas need improvement?

_____

_____

_____

Bottom Line!

A collaborative team is more than just the sum of its parts. All members will lead the effort to build trust, empower each other, engage in the shared vision, and refuel to keep the team functioning optimally.

CHAPTER KEY WORDS

Vision, Vision Statement, Collaboration, Power, Legitimate Power, Positional Power, Expert Power, Referent Power, Teams, Team Leader, Trust, Empower, Engagement

REFERENCES

1. Center for Creative Leadership. *Addressing the Leadership Gap in Healthcare.* https://www.ccl.org/articles/white-papers/addressing-the-leadership-gap-in-healthcare

2. Schaefer HG, Helmreich RL, Scheidegger D. Human factors and safety in emergency medicine. *Resuscitation.* 1994;28(3):221-225.

3. Flin R, Winter J, Cakil Sarac MR. Human factors in patient safety: review of topics and tools. *World Health.* 2009;2.

4. Carayon P, Wood K. Patient safety: the role of human factors and systems engineering. *Stud Health Technol Inform.* 2010;153:23-46.

5. Kouzes JM, Posner BZ. *The Leadership Challenge: How to Make Extraordinary Things Happen in Organizations.* 6th ed. Somerset, NJ: John Wiley & Sons, Incorporated; 2017.

6. Barker AM, Sullivan DTaylor, Emery MJ. *Leadership Competencies for Clinical Managers: The Renaissance of Transformational Leadership.* Sudbury, MA: Jones and Bartlett; 2006.

7. Fisher K, Rayner S, Belgard W. *Tips for Teams: A Ready Reference for Solving Common Team Problems.* New York, NY: McGraw-Hill; 1995.

Case Study: Crafting a Shared Vision to Lead Others

The clinic manager asked Louise and 3 of her colleagues to develop an exercise program for the clinic. The clinic manager told Louise to have the program developed within 3 months, and to start marketing it as soon as they decided how the program would be structured. The clinic manager also told Louise that she wanted all 4 of the team members to be directly involved with all aspects of developing and running this program. Louise emailed her colleagues to schedule their first team meeting. After multiple emails, they found a meeting date and time that worked for everyone on the team.

Louise had not worked directly with these colleagues on a small team before, and she was not sure how they would work together. Louise hoped that everyone would be willing to share the workload to develop this program productively, and recognized that everyone was very busy with other clinic responsibilities. Because of the imminent program deadline, she knew that it would be important for them to figure out how to work together quickly. As Louise prepared for this first team meeting, she considered using 2 approaches:

1. Approach 1: Louise would assume the team leader role and use a directive or authoritative leadership style. She would tell the team members what the clinic manager wanted, and would divide and delegate the tasks and responsibilities evenly among the 4 team members. She would generate this list of to-dos by herself and bring it to the meeting. Louise would schedule a weekly team meeting, and they would use this meeting time to check in on progress being made on each task. This approach meant that each person on the team had to work independently on the assigned tasks and had to show clear progress each week.

2. Approach 2: Louise would assume the team leader role initially to facilitate the process, and would use a participative leadership style. She would tell the team members what the clinic manager wanted, and would suggest that they use this first meeting to craft a shared vision for the exercise program. After brainstorming together, Louise would ask how they wanted to divide up the tasks and responsibilities, how often and when they wanted to meet, and how they wanted to use their meeting times (ie, to do work together, or as progress check-ins). Also, Louise would ask if they all wanted to share the team leadership responsibility, or if one volunteer was willing to assume the team leader role. This collaborative approach meant that everyone could select assignments that used their strengths, independently work on the assigned tasks, and commit to make progress each week.

From this case description, compare the approaches to teamwork by assessing the strengths and weaknesses of each approach. If you were a team member, which approach would work best for you, and why?

8.   Tuckman BW. Developmental sequence in small groups. *Psychol Bull.* 1965;63(6):384.

9.   Johnson D, Johnson F. *Joining Together: Group Theory & Group Skills.* 10th ed. Upper Saddle River, NJ: Pearson-Prentice Hall; 2009.

10. Adams K. *What Characteristics Are Necessary to Make a Self-Directed Team Work?* Small Business - Chron.com. http://smallbusiness.chron.com/characteristics-necessary-make-selfdirected-team-work-16064.html.   Published 2015. Accessed October 30, 2018.

11. Gratton L, Erickson TJ. Eight ways to build collaborative teams. *Harv Bus Rev.* 2007;85(11):100.

12. Collaboration. In: *Cambridge English Dictionary.* https://dictionary.cambridge.org/us/dictionary/english/collaboration. Accessed October 30, 2018.

13. Hackman J. *Six Common Misperceptions About Teamwork*. Boston, MA: Harvard Business Review; 2011.

14. DeBono E. *Six Thinking Hats*. New York, NY: Little Brown and Company; 1999.

15. Heinemann GD, Farrell MP, Schmitt MH. Groupthink theory and research: implications for decision making in geriatric health care teams. *Educ Gerontol Int Q*. 1994;20(1):71-85.

16. Lencioni P. *The Five Dysfunctions of a Team: A Leadership Fable*. 1st ed. San Francisco, CA: Jossey-Bass; 2002.

17. Robbins S. *Essentials of Organizational Behavior*. 11th ed. Upper Saddle River, NJ: Pearson-Prentice Hall; 2005.

18. Janis IL. *Groupthink: Psychological Studies of Policy Decisions and Fiascoes*. 2nd ed. New York, NY: Houghton Mifflin; 1982.

19. Covey SMR. *The SPEED of TRUST: The One Thing That Changes Everything*. New York, NY: Simon & Schuster; 2006.

20. Northouse PG. *Introduction to Leadership: Concepts and Practice*. Thousand Oaks, CA: SAGE Publications; 2017.

21. Cheese Peter, Thomas RJ, Craig E. *The Talent Powered Organization: Strategies for Globalization, Talent Management, and High Performance*. London, UK: Kogan Page; 2008.

22. Schaufeli WB, Salanova M, González-Romá V, Bakker AB. The measurement of engagement and burnout: a two sample confirmatory factor analytic approach. *J Happiness Stud*. 2002;3(1):71-92.

23. Schaufeli WB, Bakker AB, Salanova M. The measurement of work engagement with a short questionnaire: a cross-national study. *Educ Psychol Meas*. 2006;66(4):701-716.

24. Gallup, Inc. *State of the American Workplace*. https://news.gallup.com/reports/178514/state-american-workplace.aspx. Accessed October 30, 2018.

25. Gallup, Inc. *State of the American Workplace: Employee Engagement Insights for US Business Leaders*. http://www.gallup.com/poll/165269/worldwide-employees-engaged-work.aspx.

26. Loehr J, Schwartz T. *The Power of Full Engagement: Managing Energy, Not Time, Is the Key to High Performance and Personal Renewal*. New York, NY: Free Press; 2003.

27. The Energy Project. *The Energy Project*. https://theenergyproject.com. Accessed October 30, 2018.

28. "Are You Leading With Your Best Energy?" *Human Performance Institute*. https://energyprofile.perfprog.com/free. Accessed October 30, 2018.

29. Covey SR. *The 7 Habits of Highly Effective People: Restoring the Character Ethic*. First Fireside edition. New York, NY: Fireside Book; 1990.

SUGGESTED READINGS

Johnson DW, Johnson FP. *Joining Together: Group Theory & Group Skills*. 10th ed. Upper Saddle River, NJ: Pearson-Prentice Hall; 2009.

Lencioni P. *The Five Dysfunctions of a Team*. San Francisco, CA: Jossey-Bass; 2002.

Loehr J, Schwartz T. *The Power of Full Engagement: Managing Energy, Not Time, Is the Key to High Performance and Personal Renewal*. New York, NY: Free Press; 2003.

Leading Diversity
Becoming an Inclusive Leader

Jill Black, PT, DPT, EdD

*I believe that diversity brings new solutions to an ever-changing environment,
and that sameness is not only uninteresting but limiting.*

— *Gene Griessman, PhD, author of* Lincoln Speaks to Leaders

CHAPTER OBJECTIVES

- Articulate the depth and breadth of diversity.
- Describe the many ways that diversity impacts teams.
- Identify ways to address diversity in health care practice.
- Identify and locate resources useful in promoting a healthy work and health care practice that supports and embraces diversity.

Green-Wilson J, Zeigler S, eds.
Learning to Lead in Physical Therapy (pp 115-132).
© 2020 Taylor & Francis Group.

Leadership Vignette

Eileen C. Bach, PT, DPT, MEd

Many opportunities exist to model diversity behavior including encounters in person, by email, or through telephone conversations with patients, therapy staff, and professional colleagues. For example, as a leader, I strive to keep all possible holidays in mind when scheduling meetings or events, offer meeting food that respects dietary restrictions, ask patients or staff to "tell me what works for you—what makes you comfortable," and make efforts to be transparent in my thinking and planning. I may be an optimist, but I believe just one person can make a huge impact. That one person can be at any level; as a leader, I strive to make meaningful impacts—even through small daily actions such as my phone greeting or a thank you note summarizing an encounter. I think most of us can name at least one person who has impacted our lives, either personally or professionally, and who we remember years later. Although impact does not need to be profound each and every time, one person can make the inroad to meaningfulness. Just observing a leader or mentor managing diversity issues in a positive, proactive manner can impact actions that mirror the behavior in subsequent encounters.

I am fortunate to live and work in one of the most diverse cities in the United States, so I get to be exposed to diverse people, food, and situations every day. I have great leadership support where I work, with cultural programs to meet diverse needs in care delivery and ongoing development training opportunities for team members and management. One leadership challenge is staying abreast of all team members and not assuming knowledge and skills are present and in use consistently. Therefore, I find that we have to train and re-train or cover topics repeatedly for our large, ever-evolving team. I have learned that repetition matters!

It is important to keep cultural competence front and center, along with clinical excellence, evidenced-based care and outcomes, customer service, regulatory compliance, effectiveness, efficiency, and so many more essential items. Understanding and being skilled in diversity is at the core of good customer service, care delivery, and teamwork. My company has an immensely diverse staff, and these colleagues also bring their own real-world experiences to the process of learning about diversity, which helps make any discussion more authentic. I have also learned to be open to exploring diversity; self-awareness leads to more knowledge, which, if used, leads to more skills. Diversity is an amazingly broad domain covering gender, ethnicity, origin, language, religion, age, educational levels, disability, and even a patient's perception of illness, treatment, or pain is part of diversity. You can enhance your diversity leadership skills any time you can engage in access to and advice from diverse groups. Having cross-cultural encounters helps maintain cultural competencies and keep them relevant.

DEFINING DIVERSITY: FRAMING THE CONTEXT

Diversity is always present across teams and the many ongoing interactions the health care leader encounters. People may view diversity to refer mainly to ethnic or racial backgrounds. Although differences in ethnicity and race are apparent and certainly contribute to an individual's experience and potential barriers during interactions, diversity extends to gender, sexual orientation, religious beliefs, marital and parental status, and more. All of these dimensions of diversity in some combination influence the interactions and the collective cultures and subcultures in which people function.

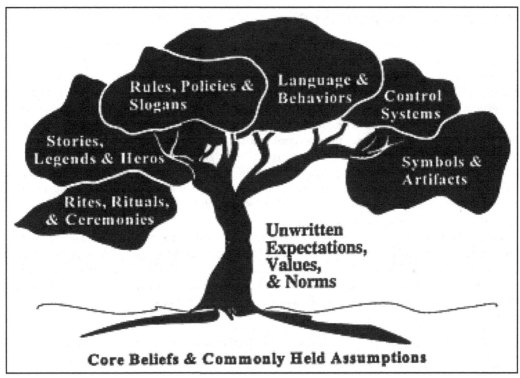

Figure 7-1. Cultural indicator tree model. (Reprinted with permission from Cultural Indicator Tree Model, US Army Business Transformation Knowledge Center. Available at http://www.comminit.com/global/content/cultural-indicator-tree-model. Accessed February 3, 2018.)

Effective leaders establish and develop relationships with individuals, and diversity and culture impact these relationships in many ways. To frame diversity further, think about *culture* as referring to the common experiences shared by individuals within a particular group, organization, or community, and then realize that each individual belongs to many cultures and subcultures (or cultures within cultures) at the same time. At this point, it becomes important to consider the influence these cultures have on shaping the way these diverse individuals view, interpret, and understand the world. Many characteristics of culture are not overtly apparent, but instead are deeply rooted and invisible. Culture has been likened to a tree in which the trunk, branches, and leaves are the most visible manifestations of culture, while the roots are the invisible elements (Figure 7-1).[1]

In this model, based on the visual image of a tree, the leaves visibly indicate the culture of a particular group, organization, or community. The trunk and branches indicate the unwritten expectations, values, and norms. The roots are core beliefs and commonly held assumptions.[1] Therefore, leaders who learn to lead by embracing and understanding the influence that all visible and invisible aspects of diversity and culture have in different situations may be able to capitalize on the advantages of diversity while leading diverse teams.

A-HA! – YOUR ROOTS

Refer to Figure 7-1. What are some of the invisible cultural traits in <u>your</u> tree roots?

_____

_____

_____

Diversity and Self-Reflection

The first and most important challenge for you as you learn to lead is to understand yourself and those aspects of diversity that you bring to the interaction and environment. The tendency is for individuals to notice the differences in others but not be aware of their own diversity, culture, and perceptions that influence and form their view of any situation. Individuals must self-reflect and self-explore to better understand the unique characteristics they bring to their leadership perspectives. Not doing so risks empowering the concepts of ethnocentrism and cultural imposition. Larry Purnell defines *ethnocentrism* as "the universal tendency of individuals to believe that their ways of thinking and behaving are the only good, proper, and right ways of thinking and behaving."[2(p23)] A key word is *universal*. Naturally, people tend to think that their way is the right way because it is the way that is most comfortable to them. The effective leader will recognize that all members of the team naturally default to ethnocentric tendencies and will help team members hear and seek to understand other perspectives, styles, and worldviews.

Left unchecked, ethnocentrism can lead to cultural imposition. In the 2006 Lattanzi and Purnell text, *cultural imposition* is defined as "the intrusive application of the majority group's cutural view upon individuals and families."[2(p15),3] Cultural imposition is often unconscious and yet can lead to major misunderstanding, miscommunication, and/or breakdown of the team/therapeutic relationship. Therefore, self-exploration and understanding of each individual's culture are essential components of being an effective leader.

A-HA! – EXAMINE YOUR BIAS

Take a few minutes to answer the following questions.
In what way might your own ethnocentrism impede your effectiveness as a leader?

_____
_____
_____

In what way might you knowingly or unknowingly practice cultural imposition?

_____
_____
_____

Diversity and Cultural Characteristics

Cultural consciousness includes variant cultural characteristics. According to Purnell,[4] variant cultural characteristics include age, generation, nationality, race, color, gender, religion, educational status, socioeconomic status, occupation, political beliefs, urban vs rural residence, enclave identity, marital status, parental status, physical characteristics, sexual orientation, gender issues, health literacy, and reason for migration (eg, sojourner immigrant asylee, or undocumented status).

With the exception of religion and age, some characteristics of culture are largely unchangeable and shape a person's understanding of the world from an early age. In many cases, early religious affiliation continues to affect a person even if the person chooses to abandon the affiliation. Although people age, they cannot change their age no matter where they are in life's continuum. Other characteristics of culture—such as socioeconomic status, length of time away from country of origin, educational status, occupation, military status, urban vs rural residence, marital status, parental status, physical characteristics, sexual orientation, and women's issues—are likely to change, adjust, and shape who people are throughout their lifetime.

A-HA! – CHARACTERISTICS OF CULTURE

What are the characteristics of culture that you, as an individual learning to lead, need to consider?

_____

_____

_____

Activity 7-1: Diagnose Your Cultural Intelligence

Cultural intelligence (CQ) is somewhat related to the concept of emotional intelligence discussed in Chapter 2. A person with high CQ can isolate the behavior of an individual or group from those in which all people and all groups would tend to exhibit; those distinctive to a particular person or group; and those who are neither universal nor unique.

The following statements in Table 7-1[5] represent a sample taken from a CQ assessment, reflecting facets of CQ—including physical CQ and emotional/motivational CQ—that may help identify growth areas for individuals needing to develop their CQ.

Diversity and Subcultures

Shared secondary characteristics often connect or bond us to others with similar secondary characteristics and represent a subculture.[3] Great commonalities might be found from shared secondary characteristics that bridge diversity in primary characteristics. For example, women who have undergone treatment for breast cancer span many cultures, and yet the shared experience of enduring breast cancer treatment results in a common bond—a subculture. Likewise, the interaction and shared experience among first-line supervisors—or formal leaders at the same level of responsibility within a health care system—also represents a subculture based on rank and status.[6] Physical therapists and occupational therapists represent subcultures within an established rehabilitation team because the professionals practice differently, have been trained differently, and have acquired a certain identity in practicing their professions.

A-HA! – SUBCULTURES

What are the subcultures that you, as an individual learning to lead, need to consider?

_____

_____

_____

Although the US culture is largely individualistic, many other cultures are more collectivistic, in which the interdependence of the group is valued.[3] Individuals identifying with a collectivistic culture are more likely to place a higher value on the group, whereas individuals who identify with an individualistic culture are more likely to place a higher value on the individual. These paradigms or

TABLE 7-1. CULTURAL INTELLIGENCE ASSESSMENT	
Directions: Use the scale to the right to rate the extent to which you agree with the following statements.	1 = Strongly Disagree 2 = Disagree 3 = Neutral 4 = Agree 5 = Strongly Agree
1. It is easy for me to change my body language (eg, eye contact or posture) to match people from a different culture.	
2. I can alter my expression when a cultural encounter requires it.	
3. I modify my speech style (eg, tone) to match people from a different culture.	
4. I easily change the way I act when a cross-cultural encounter seems to require it.	
PHYSICAL CQ TOTAL = YOUR SCORE 1 THROUGH 4 /4	
5. I have confidence that I can deal well with people from a different culture.	
6. I am certain that I can make friends with people whose cultural backgrounds are different from mine.	
7. I can adapt to the lifestyle of a different culture with relative ease.	
8. I am confident that I can deal with a cultural situation that's unfamiliar.	
EMOTIONAL/MOTIVATIONAL CQ TOTAL = YOUR SCORE 5 THROUGH 8 /4	
For both sub-scores, an average of less than 3 indicates an area for growth, while an average of 4.5 or higher indicates a CQ strength.	

Reprinted with permission from Earley PC, Mosakowski E. Cultural intelligence. *Harv Bus Rev.* 2004;82(10):139-146.

perspectives will influence many behaviors. Table 7-2[2] provides examples of behavioral traits associated with individualism and collectivism.

Activity 7-2: Are You More Individualistic or More Collectivistic in Your Behaviors?

Listed in Table 7-3[2] are 8 statements that may or may not reflect how you behave within your relationships. Review the sample list of items in Table 7-2, and for each item, determine whether you are more strongly individualistic or collectivistic. Identify where you fall on the scale for each item.

Bottom Line!

Learning to lead others involves understanding and adapting approaches for individuals of all cultures and backgrounds. Just as with all other leadership skills, the process toward effectiveness begins with leading yourself.

TABLE 7-2. EXAMPLES OF BEHAVIORAL TRAITS ASSOCIATED WITH INDIVIDUALISTIC CULTURAL TRAITS VERSUS COLLECTIVISTIC CULTURAL TRAITS

INDIVIDUALISM (THE INDIVIDUAL)	COLLECTIVISM (THE GROUP)
Doing or achieving (task-oriented)	"Being" or personal growth (non–task-related)
Independence	Interdependence
Assigns individual credit and blame	Group shares credit and blame
Time over human interaction	Human interaction over time
Characterized by informality in interactions	Characterized by formality in interactions
Respect for individuality	Respect for authority
Communication is direct (low context)	Communication is indirect (high context)
Common sense and change	Order and tradition

Reprinted with permission from Lattanzi JB, Purnell LD. *Developing Cultural Competence in Physical Therapy Practice.* Philadelphia, PA: F.A. Davis Co.; 2006.

TABLE 7-3. INDIVIDUALIST OR COLLECTIVIST SELF-ASSESSMENT

INDIVIDUALISTIC			COLLECTIVISTIC		
Doing or achieving (task-oriented)			*"Being" or personal growth (non–task-related)*		
1	2	3	4		5
Independence			*Interdependence*		
1	2	3	4		5
Assigns individual credit and blame			*Group shares credit and blame*		
1	2	3	4		5
Time over human interaction			*Human interaction over time*		
1	2	3	4		5
Characterized by informality in interactions			*Characterized by formality in interactions*		
1	2	3	4		5
Respect for individuality			*Respect for authority*		
1	2	3	4		5
Communication is direct (low context)			*Communication is indirect (high context)*		
1	2	3	4		5
Common sense and change			*Order and tradition*		
1	2	3	4		5

Reprinted with permission from Lattanzi JB, Purnell LD. *Developing Cultural Competence in Physical Therapy Practice.* Philadelphia, PA: F.A. Davis Co.; 2006.

Introducing a Model for Cultural Competence in Health Care Services

The American Physical Therapy Association (APTA) describes *cultural competence* as "a set of congruent behaviors, attitudes, and policies that come together in a system, agency, or among professionals and enable that system, agency, or those professionals to work effectively in cross-cultural situations."[7,8] The American Occupational Therapy Association (AOTA) describes *cultural competence* as the process of actively developing and practicing appropriate, relevant, and sensitive strategies and skills in interacting with culturally different persons.[9]

One model, developed by Josepha Campinha-Bacote, can be used to help individuals understand the process of cultural competence. Dr. Campinha-Bacote describes a 5-step model for the process of cultural competence in the delivery of health care services, and this model is equally applicable for those leading in a culturally diverse climate.[10]

The 5 steps include:

1. Cultural awareness
2. Cultural knowledge
3. Cultural skill
4. Cultural encounter
5. Cultural desire

The first step focuses on *cultural awareness*, which means that individuals need to be aware of their own culture and professional background. In this way, individuals can reflect upon their potential biases and the perspectives they bring to the context and interaction.

Cultural knowledge is the second step and involves learning about and understanding cultures. This does not mean memorizing a list of characteristics for all cultural groups as this would be impractical and potentially destructive, but rather obtaining an understanding of cultures. Just as intercultural variations exist among cultural groups, intracultural variations exist as well. Not everyone from the same culture is going to adhere to the same cultural norms. Essentially, humans are an amalgam of cultures, with many persons and experiences shaping who they are. Having a sense of cultures helps a leader to identify potential places of conflict that might warrant further investigation. For example, to understand that direct eye contact is deemed offensive in some cultures might cue the leader to consider that a team member or a patient/client reluctant to make eye contact is acting out of respect rather than possible disinterest.

The third step in Campinha-Bacote's model is the development of *cultural skill.*, which she describes as "the ability to conduct a cultural assessment to collect relevant cultural data regarding the client's (or team member's) presenting problem as well as accurately conducting a culturally-based physical assessment in a culturally-sensitive manner."[10(p49)] Cultural skill may also refer to applying the best leadership practices in providing culturally appropriate, effective communication to build relationships with team members as well.

The fourth and fifth steps shift from knowledge and skill to attitude and motivation. *Cultural encounter* is the fourth step, whereby the professional embraces interactions with individuals of cultures. The fifth step, *cultural desire*, represents the mindset of the professional or leader to want to embrace and engage effectively with diverse team members.[10]

Bottom Line!

Determining a consistent definition and model for cultural competence can assist those learning to lead and their followers in having a foundational understanding of the vision for effectiveness in cultural competence.

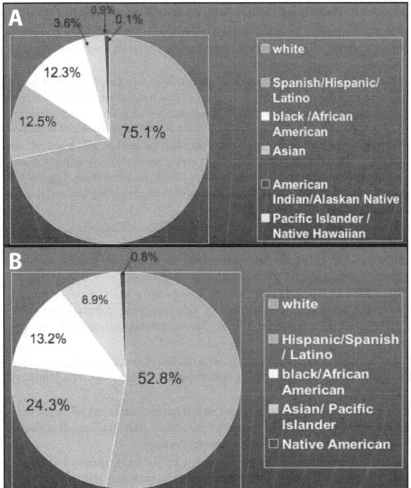

Figure 7-2. US Census Data: National Population by Race United States 2010. (Reprinted with permission from US Census Bureau, 2010 Census Data. Available at: https://www.census.gov/data/ datasets/ 2010/demo/popest/ modified-race-data-2010.html. Accessed February 3, 2018.)

DIVERSITY IN HEALTH CARE

Health professionals today will likely encounter diversity as a student, working alongside colleagues, and within the larger health care systems. They also will encounter diversity among their clients, their families, and the communities in which they serve. In Figure 7-2, the distribution of the population in the United States, based on the US Census Bureau 2010 Census data, reinforces this point.[11]

With diligent consideration and appreciation for the differences among the workforce and society, the presence of diversity can lead organizations and physical therapist practices to flourish. Just as discussed with diversity within a team in Chapter 6, diversity in health care in general can stimulate a productive breadth and depth of perspectives, innovations, and solutions. The presence of diversity is needed to broaden and enhance the group dynamics and group effectiveness in practice, and a leader is wise to ensure adequate diversity of thoughts, beliefs, cultures, and mindsets to become effective in working toward the group's shared vision.

Activity 7-3: Examine Resources for Establishing a Culturally Competent Practice

Many valuable resources are available to assist in the establishment of a culturally competent practice. Take a moment to locate the following, as well as conducting your own search, to familiarize yourself with what is available:

- The Joint Commission has reports including the 2007 report, *Hospitals, Language, and Culture: A Snapshot of the Nation*, and the 2010 roadmap, *Advancing Effective Communication, Cultural Competence, and Patient-and Family-Centered Care*. This latter report guides health care organizations on paths of quality, safety, and equity.[13] In 2011, the Joint Commission put out a field guide for creating a welcoming and inclusive environment for the lesbian, gay, bisexual, and transgender community. Connecting to the most recent online versions of these reports is an ideal way to stay up-to-date with the current information. Check out the website, http://www. jointcommission.org, for the latest on accreditation standards related to culturally and linguistically appropriate health care.
- The US Health & Human Services Office of Minority Health Cultural Competency site offers valuable resources related to cultural competence and health disparities, as well as the National Standards for Culturally and Linguistically Appropriate Services (CLAS) in Health Care. Check out the website at https://www.thinkculturalhealth.hhs.gov/clas/standards.
- Also on the HHS Office of Minority Health Cultural Competency Site is a policy timeline depicting the growth and development of addressing and promoting cultural competency and health equity. The timeline is available at https://www.thinkculturalhealth.hhs.gov/clas/ health-equity-timeline.
- The Health & Human Services Office of Minority Health has an "Action Plan to Reduce Racial and Ethnic Health Disparities" available at https://www.minorityhealth.hhs.gov/npa/templates/ content.aspx?lvl=1&lvlid=33&ID=285.
- XCulture Cross Cultural Health Care Program, available at http://xculture.org/, offers resources including a report entitled, "Reflections on the CLAS Standards: Best Practices, Innovations and Horizons." It also offers cultural competency training programs.
- The Center for the Health Professions out of the University of California (https://healthforce. ucsf.edu/) is committed to helping health care organizations and providers improve their ability to meet CLAS standards. It offers resources including *Toward Culturally Competent Care: A Toolbox for Teaching Communication Strategies*.
- The National Center for Cultural Competence at Georgetown University for Child and Human Development (https://nccc.georgetown.edu/) offers resources including the *Cultural Competence Health Practitioner Assessment*.
- The Boston Healing Landscape Project (https://www.bumc.bu.edu/gms/maccp/about/boston-healing-landscape-project/) offers cultural competency in US health care best practice recommendations with examples and resources.

Bottom Line!

An effective health care leader is wise to explore practical means of creating an environment in which diversity enhances the effectiveness of all interactions. To accomplish this, individuals must seek a greater understanding of diversity and its potential impact in all key areas.

Box 7-1

THE NATIONAL STANDARDS FOR CULTURALLY AND LINGUISTICALLY APPROPRIATE SERVICES IN HEALTH CARE

Principal Standard

Standard 1: Provide effective, equitable, understandable, and respectful quality care and services that are responsive to diverse cultural health beliefs and practices, preferred languages, health literacy, and other communication needs.

Governance, Leadership, and Workforce

Standard 2: Advance and sustain organizational governance and leadership that promotes CLAS and health equity through policy, practices, and allocated resources.

Standard 3: Recruit, promote, and support a culturally and linguistically diverse governance, leadership, and workforce that are responsive to the population in the service area.

Standard 4: Educate and train governance, leadership, and workforce in culturally and linguistically appropriate policies and practices on an ongoing basis.

(continued)

EMBRACE DIVERSITY AND INCLUSIVENESS AND EMPOWER CULTURALLY COMPETENT CARE

In the health care arena, the concern for leading a diverse team extends beyond the immediate team dynamics to the creation of a culture that empowers the team to deliver culturally competent care to the diverse communities it serves. National standards and mandates have been implemented to guide and direct health care organizations in the provision of culturally competent care.

The 2 guiding standards that will be reviewed in this chapter are The National Standards for Culturally and Linguistically Appropriate Services,[12] and the recommendations from the Joint Commission.[13] The effective leader must know these mandates and equip a team to uphold them in a concerned and caring manner. In addition, the effective leader may have opportunities to influence the larger organizational culture by helping shape mission statements, diversity statements, strategic plans, policies and procedures, and the allocation of resources.

The National Culturally and Linguistically Appropriate Services Standards in Health Care

The CLAS standards were first released by the Office of Minority Affairs of the US Department of Health & Human Services in 2001. They were revised in 2013 to advance health equity, improve quality, and help eliminate health care disparities by establishing a plan for individuals as well as health and health care organizations to implement culturally and linguistically appropriate services.[12]

The intent of the CLAS standards is "to advance health equity, improve quality and help eliminate health care disparities."[12] These 15 enhanced standards include a comprehensive series of guidelines that serves as a blueprint to inform, guide, and facilitate practices related to culturally and linguistically appropriate health care services (Box 7-1).[12] The CLAS standards are not enforced but serve as a guide for accrediting bodies such as the Joint Commission. Its website provides a tracking, by state, for implementation activity around the CLAS standards.

Box 7-1 (CONTINUED)

THE NATIONAL STANDARDS FOR CULTURALLY AND LINGUISTICALLY APPROPRIATE SERVICES IN HEALTH CARE

Communication and Language Assistance

Standard 5: Offer language assistance to individuals who have limited English proficiency and/or other communication needs, at no cost to them, to facilitate timely access to all health care and services.

Standard 6: Inform all individuals of the availability of language assistance services clearly and in their preferred language, verbally and in writing.

Standard 7: Ensure the competence of individuals providing language assistance, recognizing that the use of untrained individuals and/or minors as interpreters should be avoided.

Standard 8: Provide easy-to-understand print and multimedia materials and signage in the languages commonly used by the populations in the service area.

Engagement, Continuous Improvement, and Accountability

Standard 9: Establish culturally and linguistically appropriate goals, policies, and management accountability, and infuse them throughout the organization's planning and operations.

Standard 10: Conduct ongoing assessments of the organization's CLAS-related activities and integrate CLAS-related measures into measurement and continuous quality improvement activities.

Standard 11: Collect and maintain accurate and reliable demographic data to monitor and evaluate the impact of CLAS on health equity and outcomes and to inform service delivery.

Standard 12: Conduct regular assessments of community health assets and needs and use the results to plan and implement services that respond to the cultural and linguistic diversity of populations in the service area.

Standard 13: Partner with the community to design, implement, and evaluate policies, practices, and services to ensure cultural and linguistic appropriateness.

Standard 14: Create conflict and grievance resolution processes that are culturally and linguistically appropriate to identify, prevent, and resolve conflicts or complaints.

Standard 15: Communicate the organization's progress in implementing and sustaining CLAS to all stakeholders, constituents, and the general public.

Reprinted with permission from Office of Minority Health, US Department of Health & Human Services. *National Standards for Culturally and Linguistically Appropriate Services (CLAS) in Health Care.* Federal Register, 2013; 65(247) 80865-79.

Notice that the principal standard sets the context for health and health care organizations to "provide effective, equitable, understandable, and respectful quality care and services that are responsive to diverse cultural health beliefs and practices, preferred languages, health literacy, and other communication needs."[12]

Standards 2 through 4 are specific for governance, leadership, and workforce, encouraging the recruitment of employees (team members) from communities that represent the surrounding service area, as well as for regular cultural competency training for the workforce.

CLAS standards 5 through 8 address language access services and mandate that organizations provide language assistance at no cost to the client, at all points of contact, in a timely manner, during all hours of operation. Furthermore, the organization must inform each client of the right to language assistance access, as well as ensure that the language service provided is competent. Lastly, the standards dictate that client educational materials and signage should be available and displayed in the languages most commonly encountered in the geographic region of service.

CLAS standards 9 to 15 mandate organizational support for the provision of culturally competent care. These organizational supports call for inclusion of culturally competent care in the strategic plan, ongoing self-assessment of organizational cultural competency, and establishment of policies that are culturally and linguistically appropriate. In addition, the organizational support mandates include directives that call for the recognition and resolution of potential health care disparities. To that end, they require that health care organizations keep data records that include race, ethnicity, and spoken and written language preferences in health records; conduct community needs assessments; and become familiar with the demographic, cultural, and epidemiological profile of the local community. As the organization gathers and tracks these data, it should be seeking ways in which it might collaborate with community partners to better service the health care needs of the community.

Joint Commission Leadership Domains

The Joint Commission is an independent, not-for-profit group in the United States that oversees and manages accreditation programs for hospitals and other health care organizations. The Commission develops performance standards that deal with crucial elements of operation, such as patient care, medication safety, infection control, and consumer rights. With the CLAS standards as a backdrop, the 2007 Joint Commission Report, *Hospitals, Language and Culture: A Snapshot of the Nation*,[14] identified 6 domains for effective organizational management of diversity, including leadership, quality improvement and data, workforce, patient safety and provision of care, language services, and community engagement. The full report can be found at http://www.jointcommission.org/assets/1/6/hlc_paper.pdf.

Leadership is the first domain identified by the Joint Commission, with the recognition that organizational culture is established from the top. To that end, do formal leadership and higher-level management support diversity endeavors? Is it reflected in the organizational mission statement, strategic plan, or vision? Are funds allotted to address diversity-related issues such as payment for medical interpreter services and acquisition and tracking of community health statistics and potential disparities? Relative to this domain, it was recommended that hospital CEOs and other hospital leaders should make their commitment to culturally and linguistically appropriate care highly visible to hospital staff and patients, and that more research is needed to better understand what motivates hospital CEOs who embrace culturally and linguistically appropriate care.[14]

A-HA! – WHAT IS IN YOUR VISION?

Whether you are taking classes to become a health care professional or are already in the field, the organization you are associated with has a mission and vision (and, hopefully, a strategic plan). Ask yourself:

Do you know the mission and vision of your organization?

_____

Do these statements clearly appear to include or support diversity endeavors for the organization, or does the organization have a separate diversity statement for this purpose?

_____

What measures have been taken within the organization to promote diversity?

Bottom Line!

The effective leader must be aware of guidelines and mandates for positioning the team toward the shared vision with diversity and inclusiveness in mind. Competence in this area helps establish trust among the team, and trust that the team's leader has everyone's best interests at heart.

Leading Diversity Effectively:
Becoming an Inclusive Leader

Diversity within and among teams can yield tremendous advantages if and when the synergy and diversity of perspectives are considered and incorporated. Ultimately, leveraging diversity can lead to more effective problem solving and program development. Without a doubt, team leaders play a critical role in facilitating effective, diverse teamwork. Leaders of diverse teams create linkages and connectedness to facilitate effective interdependent work with multiple people and multiple systems.[15] These leaders help encourage flexible thinking, translate complexity, focus on delegating responsibility to team members, and work to empower the team to accomplish the assigned tasks and responsibilities. Leaders can be the role models and champions of the unique collective identity by enhancing the identity of each individual as someone who adds value.[15] The ultimate goal for the inclusive leader leading diverse teams is to create an environment in which team members value and respect one another in the midst of their diversity. The process of cultural competency development for leaders learning to lead begins with cultural awareness.[10]

Cultural awareness includes self-awareness, as well as awareness of others on the team. Individuals can develop cultural competency by acquiring awareness of their existence, sensations, thoughts, and environment, without any influence from other backgrounds.[4] Typically, because culture and related characteristics are such a part of a person's background and upbringing, it is often difficult for individuals to recognize their own diversity and how their culture and habits are different from others'. An in-depth, self-reflective cultural exploration will help identify potential challenges and barriers that might occur while leading a diverse team.

Once leaders understand their own attributes and perspectives, they can explore the cultural diversity present within the team, both the interprofessional (horizontal) and hierarchical (vertical) team, as well as the client population or communities served. As leaders explore, they should avoid negative stereotyping and overgeneralizations. Generalizations about behaviors and characteristics do not usually apply to all individuals in the group and can hinder positive group dynamics. Rather than assume team members' cultures and perspectives are a certain way, leaders can begin to explore the mindsets and viewpoints of individual team members by showing interest and respect for each unique person, leading to an increased understanding and enhanced team dynamics. Effective leaders will get to know each member of the team and seek to include their talents, strengths, and perspectives into the goals and direction of the group. As leaders work to identify, display respect, and

---

Box 7-2

A SAMPLE OF APTA'S MAJOR VALUES AND PRINCIPLES OF A CULTURALLY COMPETENT SYSTEM

- The family as defined by each culture is the primary system of support and preferred intervention.
- The system must recognize that racial and ethnic populations have to be at least bicultural, and that this status may create a unique set of issues to which the system must be equipped to respond.
- Individuals and families make different choices based on cultural forces; these choices must be considered if education/service delivery are to be helpful and appropriate.
- Practice is driven in the service delivery system by culturally preferred choices, not by culturally blind or culturally free interventions.
- Inherent in cross-cultural interactions are dynamics that must be acknowledged, adjusted to, and accepted.
- The system must sanction and, in some cases, mandate the incorporation of cultural knowledge into policymaking, education and practice.
- Cultural competence involves determining an individual or family's cultural identity and levels of acculturation and assimilation in order to more effectively apply the helping principle of "starting where the individual or family is."
- Cultural competence seeks to identify and understand the needs and help-seeking behaviors of individuals and families. Cultural competence seeks to design and implement services that are tailored or matched to the unique needs of individuals, children, and families.

Reprinted with permission from American Physical Therapy Association. *Achieving Cultural Competence: Major Values and Principles of a Culturally Competent System.* Alexandria, VA; 2007. Available at: http://www.apta.org/CulturalCompetence/Achieving/. Accessed February 3, 2018.

---

demonstrate value for the cultural differences within the team, they are creating an open and flexible environment in which diverse viewpoints and communication styles will be tolerated and flourish.

Activity 7-4: Start Leading Toward Diversity

Take steps today to get started in your quest to lead toward diversity and to leverage the strengths of cultural competence in your leadership capacity. The APTA and AOTA offer the tools listed here as options toward taking initial steps that will apply to the diverse populations you encounter all across health care:

- APTA Learning Center – "Clinical Decision-Making in Diverse Populations." This online course can found here: http://learningcenter.apta.org/student/Catalogue/CatalogueCategory.aspx?id=7790e723-af77-453a-b93e-e50d107604a3. Note, there is a charge for taking this course.
- Review APTA's perspective on "Achieving Cultural Competence" and related "Major Values and Principles of a Culturally Competent System": http://www.apta.org/CulturalCompetence/Achieving/.[7] Box 7-2[7] also has a sample of APTA's Major Values and Principles of a Culturally Competent System.

- Explore the AOTA's Cultural Competency Toolkits[16] at https://www.aota.org/Practice/Manage/Multicultural/Cultural-Competency-Tool-Kit.aspx.
- Become a Member of the Global Health Special Interest Group (SIG), part of APTA's HPA The Catalyst Section. The purpose of the Global Health SIG[17] (http://www.aptahpa.org/?page=GlobalHealthSIG) is to provide resources, information, and support to SIG, HPA The Catalyst Section, and APTA members regarding the mission to provide resources, information, and support to SIG, Section, and APTA members regarding global health, health disparities, cultural competency, disability, and service-learning in resource-limited settings. The Global Health SIG functions include the following services:
  - Providing programs and opportunities for the exchange of information related to considerations concerning culture and diversity, international and global physical therapy, and service learning
  - Serving as a direct resource to the HPA The Catalyst Section on health policy and administrative matters related to cultural and diversity considerations, including health disparities
  - Serving as a liaison to outside organizations sharing similar interests and seeking to establish networks and collaborative programs to promote culturally competent physical therapist practices
  - Collaborating with physical therapists from other countries to advance physical therapy education, exchanges, and programs
  - Encouraging physical therapy research and publication in the areas of culture and diversity considerations

Bottom Line!

"In highly complex systems, we need leaders who have skills resembling those of an accomplished orchestral conductor. Such individuals understand and interpret the score across a wide range of players. Without having extensively read the score or heard the piece before, they can, with minimal rehearsal, lead the performers to great coordinated achievement."[15(p653)]

Case Study: Diversity and Leadership

Sandra has recently been appointed to the clinical director position at an urban outpatient clinic within a large health system. She has been practicing physical therapy in the outpatient setting for 5 years and has recently participated in a leadership development program offered through her professional association.

Sandra will oversee a team of:
- 4 physical therapists
- 5 physical therapist assistants
- 3 aides
- 4 office personnel

Of the staff members, 4 are male, and 12 are female. Their ages range from 19 to 54 years. Of the 5 physical therapists, Sandra is the only one who pursued her doctorate of physical therapy degree.

Sandra will be reporting to 3 bosses within the hospital system; 2 are male and 1 is female. The outpatient and hospital center is located within an urban environment serving the urban and surrounding suburban areas. Public transportation allows for easy access from the local suburbs, attracting many suburbanites to this well-known medical center.

Imagine that you are the newest member on Sandra's team. You are new to this area and new to this organization.

- *How you would start to build relationships with other members on the team?*
- *What would you do?*
- *Would there be any interactions that would seem more difficult to initiate?*
- *Why or why not?*

In the case study, Sandra finds herself needing to lead a diverse team of staff and health care professionals, represent her team to a diverse group of interprofessional colleagues and supervisors, and create an environment in which her team can provide culturally competent health care to a diverse group of clients. She recognizes that she needs to operate and lead effectively within 3 unique communities: her immediate clinic team, the larger interprofessional team and leadership hierarchy, and the local community of clients that will be served by her clinical team. The following discussion considers how Sandra can enhance her effectiveness in leading and influencing such diverse groups.

First, to be an effective leader, Sandra must self-reflect to better understand who she is and how her approach and mindset might impact the situations she will encounter as a leader of a diverse team. Sandra must consider her own cultural characteristics that may have an influence on her approach.

Second, Sandra may be aware of some obvious cultural differences in her team, but most likely needs to unearth the invisible, less obvious roots of diversity if she is to uncover and overcome potential cultural barriers effectively. Sandra needs to avoid generalizing about group behaviors and characteristics that do not apply to all individuals within her team. Rather than assume team members' cultures and perspectives are a certain way, Sandra can begin to explore the mindsets and viewpoints of individual team members by showing interest and respect for each unique person. Sandra can be an effective leader in this discovery process by developing her own inclusive leadership style and her ability to lead as the facilitator of the group (vs assuming an authoritarian or directing leadership style). These actions will lead to an increased understanding and enhanced team dynamics. Sandra needs to identify and consider possible challenges that communication styles and leadership/followership styles might also bring to her team. Furthermore, recognition of cultural differences impacting verbal and nonverbal language will facilitate more effective communication.

Finally, within her immediate clinical setting, Sandra has a distinct mix of staff and health care professionals who share the common goal of providing optimal physical therapy service to clients in need. Identifying the common bonds that exist in team members will help Sandra establish common ground for accomplishing group goals. To accomplish this goal, she must identify the diverse backgrounds and cultural characteristics of the team members, beginning with her own culture, communication patterns, expectations, and biases. For example, Sandra recognizes that it may be helpful to intentionally identify and consider the primary and secondary characteristics of culture and subcultures that are present among her team. Sandra also needs to watch proactively for possible manifestations of secondary cultural characteristics in behaviors of all of her team members, and help her team become more aware of the impact of these behaviors on team functioning. Furthermore, Sandra may face ongoing conflict and misunderstandings arising from other sources, especially when organizational and other pressures to perform and produce as a team intensify.

CHAPTER KEY WORDS

Culture, Subculture, Ethnocentrism, Cultural Imposition, Cultural Intelligence, Diversity, Cultural Competence

REFERENCES

1. Cultural Indicator Tree Model. *US Army Business Transformation Knowledge Center*. http://www.comminit.com/global/content/cultural-indicator-tree-model. Accessed October 30, 2018.

2. Lattanzi JB, Purnell LD. *Developing Cultural Competence in Physical Therapy Practice*. Philadelphia, PA: F.A. Davis Co.; 2006.

3. Purnell LD. *Guide to Culturally Competent Health Care*. 3rd ed. Philadelphia, PA: F.A. Davis Company; 2014.

4. Purnell LD. *Transcultural Healthcare: A Culturally Competent Approach*. 4th ed. Davis Plus ebook pdf version; 2013.

5. Earley PC, Mosakowski E. Cultural intelligence. *Harv Bus Rev*. 2004;82(10):139-146.

6. Schein EH. *Organizational Culture and Leadership*. 4th ed. San Francisco, CA: Jossey-Bass; 2010.

7. American Physical Therapy Association. *Achieving Cultural Competence: Major Values and Principles of a Culturally Competent System*. http://www.apta.org/CulturalCompetence/Achieving. Published 2013. Accessed October 30, 2018.

8. Cross T, Bazron B, Dennis K, Isaacs M. *Towards A Culturally Competent System of Care*. vol 1. Washington, DC: Georgetown University Child Development Center, CASSP Technical Assistance Center; 1989.

9. Odawara E. Cultural competency in occupational therapy: beyond a cross-cultural view of practice. *Am J Occup Ther*. 2005;59:325-334.

10. Campinha-Bacote J. *The Process of Cultural Competence in the Delivery of Healthcare Services: The Journey Continues*. 5th ed. Cincinnati, OH: Transcultural C.A.R.E. Associates; 2007.

11. US Census Bureau. *2010 Census Data*. https://www.census.gov/data/datasets/2010/demo/popest/modified-race-data-2010.html. Accessed October 30, 2018.

12. Federal Register. *National Standards for Culturally and Linguistically Appropriate Services (CLAS) in Health Care*. Office of Minority Health, US Department of Health & Human Services.

13. The Joint Commission. *Advancing Effective Communication, Cultural Competence, and Patient- and Family-Centered Care: A Roadmap for Hospital for Hospitals*. Oakbrook Terrace, IL: Author; 2010.

14. The Joint Commission. *Hospitals, Language and Culture: A Snapshot of the Nation.*; 2007. http://www.jointcommission.org/assets/1/6/hlc_paper.pdf.

15. Dowton SB. Leadership in medicine: where are the leaders? *Med J Aust*. 2004;181(11/12):652.

16. American Occupational Therapy Association. *AOTA Cultural Competency Toolkit*. https://www.aota.org/Practice/Manage/Multicultural/Cultural-Competency-Tool-Kit.aspx. Accessed October 30, 2018.

17. Global Health Special Interest Group. http://www.aptahpa.org/?page=GlobalHealthSIG. Accessed October 30, 2018.

SUGGESTED READING

Purnell LD. *Culturally Competent Health Care*. 3rd ed. Philadelphia, PA: FA Davis; 2014.

8

Leading Through Conflict

Jennifer Green-Wilson, PT, MBA, EdD
Beth Danehy, MA, MS, LMFT, CEAP

*In any encounter we have a choice: we can strengthen our resentment or our understanding
and empathy. We can widen the gap between ourselves and others or lessen it.*
— *Pema Chodron, American Tibetan Buddhist*

CHAPTER OBJECTIVES

- Define *conflict*.
- Identify sources of conflict.
- Self-assess your conflict management style.
- Discuss why conflict can be perceived as "dangerous."
- Describe how conflict can be framed as a positive element in relationships.
- Examine strategies for leading through conflict.

Green-Wilson J, Zeigler S, eds.
Learning to Lead in Physical Therapy (pp 133-156).
© 2020 Taylor & Francis Group.

Leadership Vignette

Sheila K. Nicholson, PT, DPT, JD, MBA, MA

I have held many leadership roles as a volunteer and as an employee. I never consider myself an expert in leadership but always seize opportunities to learn more about it. One of the greatest challenges in any leadership role is managing and facilitating conflicts. Some conflict situations are easy to manage, while others are difficult and cannot always be managed. Thus, learning and developing the skills to both assess conflicts and recognize how they occur will serve you well in volunteer positions as well as in your professional career.

I have learned several lessons about leading through conflict. For example, an effective leader looks at all sides of the conflict situation and does not prejudge or let biases interfere. As a leader, I find that putting aside my views to look at the conflict situation objectively, and considering first what is best for the team or organization, are the most challenging parts of managing conflict. I have also learned to not take criticism personally. As a leader, I must have confidence in the decisions I make or facilitate, not by attempting to please everyone—an impossible task—but by being impartial and doing my best to resolve conflict.

CONFLICT AND LEADERSHIP

As each chapter of this book has described, effective leadership relies on establishing and maintaining relationships. Chapter 6 went one step further to describe the necessity of inviting diversity of people and thought for highly productive teams. In this chapter, the often-dreaded conversation about conflict is discussed.

The Cambridge English Dictionary describes *conflict* as an active disagreement between opposing opinions or needs.[1] Conflict is also popularly described using words such as *disharmony*, *argument*, *clash*, *tension*, *disagreement*, *struggle*, or *battle*. With these descriptors, it is no wonder that most individuals, particularly those responsible for leading a team, would want to avoid it. Making things even more challenging is the extant nature of conflict occurring at 4 distinct, and sometimes overlapping, levels including *intrapersonal conflict* (conflict within one self), *interpersonal conflict* (conflict between 2 people), *intergroup conflict* (conflict between 2 groups), and *interorganizational conflict* (conflict between 2 organizations).

On a more positive note, consider the Chinese symbol for conflict, which is composed of 2 characters: one meaning danger, and the other meaning opportunity. Conflict does contain both of these elements, although too often, our culture focuses on the danger, failing to appreciate the opportunity that constructive conflict can bring. Conflict is inevitable, and those learning to lead need to become effective in both overcoming the dangers and capitalizing on the opportunities. This chapter will discuss both aspects, starting with engaging the opportunities, and ending with identifying and overcoming the dangers.

A-HA! – YOUR PERCEPTION OF CONFLICT

Do you perceive conflict to be mostly dangerous, mostly opportunity-filled, or a little of both? Why?

_____

_____

_____

What is an example of a conflict that had a high degree of danger?

_____

_____

_____

What is an example of a conflict that had a high degree of opportunity?

_____

_____

_____

How do you feel your past experiences with conflict have shaped your current attitudes for conflict engagement and resolution?

_____

_____

_____

Embracing Different Conflict Perspectives

Leaders can become influential in transforming conflict by developing an awareness of how they tend to name and frame conflict, and how their mindset may be influenced by factors such as their own interests, needs, and values; their education, life, and work experiences; their formal and informal roles in teams and organizations; their profession; and their relationships. As different factors have formed every person's individual viewpoints and approaches to conflict, having a greater understanding of the types of perspectives about conflict itself is foundational. Table 8-1: Categories of Conflict Perspectives details the background for how individuals may perceive conflict and their reactions to it.

A-HA! – CONFLICT PERSPECTIVE CATEGORY

Which of the categories listed in Table 8-1 best resembles your natural tendency to view conflict?

_____

_____

_____

Which of the categories do you feel would be most valuable for effective leadership?

_____

_____

_____

TABLE 8-1. CATEGORIES OF CONFLICT PERSPECTIVES	
PERSPECTIVE OF CONFLICT	**DESCRIPTION**
Human relations or behavioral perspective	Conflict is seen as constructive and beneficial. Conflict is seen as a natural part of groups and organizations. Conflict is a fundamental part of the human experience. Conflict exists and must be tolerated.
Traditional perspective	Conflict must be resolved. Conflict is seen as uncomfortable, dysfunctional, negative, and irrational. Conflict may be caused by a lack of trust, poor communication, or a failure to be accountable to the needs of others.
Interactionist perspective	Conflict is encouraged because it is seen as one of the forces that keeps individuals and groups viable and creative. A lack of conflict means that people and organizations may become stagnant and slow to respond.
Relational perspective	Conflict is viewed as a breakdown in the relationship itself. Conflict may lead to a strengthened relationship if opportunities to transform conflict are explored and allowed.

Accepting Conflict

Because conflict is entrenched in all human interactions, resolving conflict may realistically only be an aspiration.[2] Conflict may *never* truly or completely be resolved. Therefore, in most cases, and despite the challenge, living with conflict and participating in it constructively may be a more realistic goal than resolving it. It may be more realistic to accept the role that enduring conflict has in day-to-day living and to learn how to stay engaged or reside in conflict in constructive and effective ways, rather than trying to resolve it or settle it.[2] Moreover, Mayer suggests that people's satisfaction with their lives and their relationships may be more determined by their ability to stay (tolerate/accept) and evolve with enduring conflicts than by the success they have in resolving these conflicts. That is, when they engage in conflict productively, people and relationships may have opportunities to make significant and transformational changes.

Bottom Line!

Leaders learning to lead need to frame conflict in a positive way, considering its inevitable and extensive link to establishing and maintaining the relationships needed for effective leadership. Your perspective on conflict will influence your actions, but a new perspective can be learned and cultivated through engagement and practice.

CONFLICT: OPPORTUNITY FOR GROWTH

Conflict can be positive! Conflict can improve the quality of decisions, release tensions that may be overt or covert, stimulate creative thinking and innovation, spark interest, and hopefully, encourage self-reflection and self-improvement. Conflict may also help to combat groupthink, or the awkward phenomenon of approaching problems as matters dealt only by consensus of the group rather than by individuals acting independently, as discussed in Chapter 6. Conflict may be transformational because it encourages growth, change, learning, and a deeper understanding of self and others. In some cases, conflict may strengthen relationships by building greater confidence in a person's ability to work with and through differences, and by building greater trust within the relationship itself.

Imagine how different a transforming conflict experience might be if it came from individuals, as leaders, who were willing to truly understand the needs and interests of others as well as their own, instead of approaching conflict from fear, risk, or from feelings of a potential loss or anger. When leaders make room at the table for everybody's needs to co-exist and to find ways to value all of these needs in some way, then they may arrive at a different set of approaches or resolutions to conflict that are sustainable. Trust and empathy, already discussed in this book, play a critical role in a collaborative process during conflict.

Establishing Trust

Reviewing from Chapter 2, trust develops in relationships when motives are clear, honest, transparent, and based on mutual benefit. Lack of trust among one or both parties prevents any dynamic, such as conflict, from changing, either because the parties choose not to change or because they are unable to change. In his book *The SPEED of TRUST*, Stephen M. R. Covey identifies how to see, speak, and behave in ways that establish trust.[3] The premise behind this framework is that if you change your mindset or the way you see a situation, this may change your actions or your behavior and, ultimately, your results. Behaviors such as demonstrating respect, creating transparency, clarifying expectations, practicing accountability, listening first, and keeping commitments were found to be common in high-trust leader-follower relationships.[3] Regarding conflict, keep in mind from Chapter 5 how the presence or absence of trust may impact communication styles and, ultimately, relationships that leaders can develop. For example, when trust is low, then the style of communication may be characterized by defensiveness or protectiveness, whereas when trust is high, the style of communication may be characterized by cooperative and creative synergy.[3]

Empathy

Empathy is the ability to understand and share the feelings, thoughts, or attitudes of another person. Empathy is a skill that may be enhanced through practice, and it can be empowering. When individuals understand another person's perspective, it helps them analyze the situation more objectively and understand their own role in the conflict.

One way to develop empathy is to practice listening with empathy. Often, especially in situations of conflict, individuals strive to be understood or heard first. People want to make sure that others know their side of the story. Yet, rather than listening to these different sides of the story, people often prepare their own replies before it is time to reply. They typically listen with the intent to reply, and not with the intent to listen.[3] Many times, people filter everything through their own lenses and experiences, and yet proclaim, "Oh, I know how you feel. I've had that happen to me before too." Listening with empathy means that individuals listen by trying to get inside another person's frame of reference, and that they listen with their hearts as well as their ears.[3] This point is echoed by Patterson, Grenny, McMillan, and Switzler in their book, *Crucial Conversations*, in which they describe "start with the heart" as the first step toward having the conversations that deal with hard issues.[4] When you start with the heart, you not only focus on what you want, but you also consider what others want as well. The greatest danger in attempting to be empathic is to assume that you understand the other person's viewpoint. There is no way to know where another person is coming from without asking and really listening to the thoughts and feelings of the other participants in the conflict.

In his 1993 book, *Getting Past No: Negotiating Your Way from Confrontation to Cooperation*, William Ury introduces the joint problem-solving approach.[5] The point is to get the problem off of the people involved in the conflict and onto the shared problem of the parties to come to a collaborative solution. Not so ironically, this approach also identifies the first 2 steps as identifying your concerns, issues, and problems, and then identifying the other person's concerns, issues, and problems. In the planning process, you try to put yourself in the other person's shoes to anticipate the needs of the other person before you enter into the conversation. However, you make a critical mistake if you forget to ask the other parties for their thoughts, feelings, attitudes, and concerns about their side of the conflict before moving further into the conversation. That is, failure occurs when you forget to practice empathy.

Activity 8-1: Practice Empathy

In your next conflict situation, start the conversation with:

- "Can we talk about the way that you see things in this situation?"
- "What do you feel is your greatest concern on this topic?"
- "How strongly do you feel about the outcome that we reach?"

As discussed in Chapter 5, practice active listening skills during their answers. Do not interrupt. Listen, and do not respond with an immediate solution. Do not walk away until they tell you that they feel you understand their position.

While the matter may not be solved that day, at a minimum, you will have established trust with the other individual through empathic listening, which will make future conversations more productive toward a collaborative solution.

Bottom Line!

Conflict can be positive and is an opportunity to establish and build strong relationships toward leadership effectiveness! Transforming conflict requires individuals to have an awareness of self and an awareness of others, and to value both equally. Simply agreeing or seeing things the same way is not the same as making room for understanding how other people view situations, or how they express their values.

CONFLICT MANAGEMENT STYLES

Frameworks have been developed to help individuals understand how they respond to conflict or to determine their conflict management style. By gaining this information, leaders who are learning to lead can practice how they need to respond or adapt to conflict situations and can have a better understanding of others' approaches as well.

The Thomas-Kilmann Conflict Mode Instrument (TKI)[6] is commonly used to appraise an individual's approach or behavior in conflict situations. In this framework, the individual's behavior is described as varying combinations of assertiveness and cooperativeness. *Assertiveness* explains the degree to which individuals try to satisfy their own interests, whereas *cooperativeness* is the degree to which individuals try to satisfy the other person's concerns. These 2 specific dimensions of behavior are combined in various ways to identify 5 approaches of dealing with or handling conflict: competing, accommodating, avoiding, collaborating, and compromising.

According to this framework, each of the styles can be effective. The most effective style may differ depending upon the situation. Additionally, each style can be applied with differing approaches.

For example, the competing style can be implemented as a demand—applying a power-oriented, authoritarian, or win-lose approach. The goal is to win, and individuals pursue their own interests.

An individual adopting a win-lose approach views the situation as, "If I win, you lose," and, "I get my way; you don't get yours".[7] An example would be if a senior physical therapist told the rest of the team that her schedule at work could *only* be 8 am to 4 pm, Monday through Friday, because she had seniority as a therapist and also had a family that needed her to be home by 4:40 pm. This demand is a win for her because she gets a schedule that fits her needs, but it may be a loss for the other therapists who also have families, are also juggling work-life demands, and will now need to work early mornings, evenings, and Saturdays to cover the clinic's established hours of operation. Sadly, this win-lose paradigm is a common thought process in many conflict situations, reinforcing fear and danger with the notion that only one person will get what he or she wants. The competing style can also be applied using persuasiveness (eg, stating, "I think that when you hear me out, you may agree that this is an important issue.").

The opposite of the competing style is an accommodating or adapting style. Accommodating may show up as an unassertive but cooperative approach. When an accommodating style is used, individuals may neglect or sacrifice their own concerns to satisfy the concerns of another person. Accommodating might also mean that individuals give in to another person's demand or concede to another's point of view. Using the scenario described previously, an example of an accommodating style is when a therapist on the team simply accepts the senior therapist's schedule demand without challenging it or without advocating for his or her own ideal schedule. Accommodating the needs of a competitor's style reinforces the win-lose mentality because the accommodator simply gives in. However, situations may exist when the relationship outweighs an individual's interest in a given moment, and accommodation may be an appropriate style to use.

In the TKI framework,[6] the avoiding style is described as both unassertive and uncooperative. Individuals who avoid conflict may avoid the issue entirely, or sidestep issues diplomatically, postponing them for another time, or withdraw completely from situations that seem threatening or uncomfortable. An example of an avoiding style is seen when a team member (the sender) sends the physical therapist in charge of scheduling for the clinic (the scheduler) an abrasive email, and the scheduler deletes this curt email and does not respond, call, or talk to the sender. Covey would describe this approach as lose-win, a giving-in or giving-up approach, which is seen as even worse than a win-lose approach because the scheduler simply will not even engage in the conflict process.

The collaborative style is opposite from the avoiding style in that those who collaborate are both assertive and cooperative.[6] A collaborative approach to leading through conflict means that individuals attempt to work with the other person to resolve the conflict in such a way to satisfy the concerns of both sides. This style may also be viewed as the win-win approach. Collaboration involves staying engaged long enough to dig deeper into an issue to identify the underlying concerns of both individuals, and then to find alternatives that meet the concerns of both sides. In many cases, this style requires time and energy and may be best applied to situations when both the relationship and the outcome are important. An example of a collaborating style is when the physical therapist in charge of the scheduling for the clinic asks each therapist to submit their ideal schedule and to highlight any schedule restrictions or special requests they have and then works on developing a couple of options for the team to consider before implementing any scheduling changes. In this way, the team can provide input, all team members have a voice, and they decide collectively which schedule option works the best for everyone. Collaborating is an ideal conflict management style in many situations because the parties engaged in the conflict derive a solution or strategy that takes what both parties want and then synergizes these options together to develop an even better resolution.

The final style is the compromising style. This style is midway between being assertive and being cooperative, but is not always the ideal approach to managing conflict because, to compromise, both sides need to give something up. This may create an experience of lose-lose in which both parties walk away without what they wanted or needed from the process. To compromise, the objective is to find an expedient, mutually acceptable solution that partially satisfies both parties. Compromising might mean splitting the difference, conceding on certain arrangements, or seeking a quick middle-ground position to achieve certain goals and objectives. While this style can be effective when a quick resolution is needed, it does not capitalize on finding all the opportunities that the situation might bring. An example of a compromising style is when each member of the team is required to work at least one evening shift and one early morning shift per week plus one Saturday shift per month, even though each member of the team is juggling unique work-life balance and issues.

Activity 8-2: Discovering Your Conflict Management Style

TKI,[6] a conflict style inventory, measures an individual's response to conflict situations. The TKI mode instrument consists of 30 pairs of statements, and the respondent is asked to choose either A or B for each pair (forced response). The TKI uses 2 axes—assertiveness and cooperativeness—and identifies 5 styles of conflict.

Complete the TKI self-assessment online, or, if you prefer, you can complete it as a hard copy self-assessment. A cost is associated with its use. To order, visit cpp.com/products or call customer service at 1-800-624-1765.

Many other conflict management questionnaires that are not proprietary are also available on the internet. For this activity, find an online survey to determine your default conflict management style, and review your results.

Increasing Opportunity With Conflict Styles

Just as with personality styles (Chapter 1), leadership and followership styles (Chapter 3), and communication styles (Chapter 5), each individual, while a composite of the variety of styles, does tend to have more of a default style to leading through conflict. People may tend to gravitate to certain styles that are easier or more comfortable to use and, therefore, they tend to rely on them more often. According to the TKI framework,[6] when individuals learn to use each of the 5 conflict management styles at different times and in different situations, then they may become more effective at leading through all types of conflict.

For instance, the competing style may be the most useful style to use when quick, decisive action is crucial, such as in an emergency situation or when the fire alarm starts ringing and everyone must exit the clinic immediately.

An accommodating approach to conflict may be useful when there is a need to show a willingness to listen and learn from others or when a goodwill gesture is needed to maintain a cooperative relationship. For example, if an issue is more important to one person than it is to another, and if the outcome of this decision does not harm the other party, then an accommodating style may help to preserve some harmony within the relationship and avoid further disruption in the ability to work together.

Avoiding may be an appropriate way to deal with conflict when an issue is trivial in comparison to the other more important or urgent issues, there is not enough time to address the issue constructively, more time or information is needed, or angry people literally need time to cool down before they can engage in an important but less tension-filled conversation.

The collaborating style may be the most useful when a solution needs to integrate multiple perspectives to a problem, when collective buy-in is required before change (such as a large-scale schedule change) can be implemented, or when lingering, hard feelings between 2 people or between 2 groups interfere with productive work relationships.

Other times, a compromising style may be used effectively when 2 opponents with equal power are strongly committed to mutually exclusive goals, or when a temporary settlement of a complex issue is needed quickly.

A-HA! – YOUR LAST CONFLICT

The last time you faced a conflict, what was your default conflict management style?

_____

In reflection, was that the best style you could have used for that situation to maximize the opportunities of the situation? Why or why not?

_____

_____

_____

Could a collaborative style have been used, and how could this have been implemented effectively?

_____

_____

_____

Bottom Line!

How you respond to and resolve conflict, and understanding how others do the same, will be pivotal in your success as a leader.

CONFLICT: GETTING PAST DANGER

Leadership is about relationships. Relationships will bring conflict. Conflict brings both danger and opportunity. An effective leader has the skill to maximize the opportunity and minimize the danger. Dangers to be recognized that are covered next in this section include fear, anger, microaggression, bullying, and apathy. Learning the skills necessary to get past these dangers begins as all other skills in this book: through self-awareness and self-assessment.

Fear

Much of the personal danger in conflict is engendered and expressed in the emotion of fear: fear of losing what you want, fear of damaging the relationships in the conflict (hurting people's feelings), fear of not having what it takes to make it through the conflict situation, fear of not being an effective enough leader, and so on. In Lencioni's book, *The Five Dysfunctions of a Team*,[8] fear of conflict is the second dysfunction. Lencioni makes the point that great relationships are built on the ability to disagree, even passionately at times, and to know that you can recover from that, and it can get better. The best teams are those who have the trust in each other, and who understand that conflict is necessary and valued. Personal fear of conflict is going to be emotionally uncomfortable whether an individual faces the conflict or avoids it, and avoiding a conflict is much more dangerous—personally and professionally—than facing it. Leaders learning to lead need to embrace the risk of conflict and be prepared to reframe the danger, including personal fear.

A-HA! – FEAR OF CONFLICT

Review your results from Activity 8-2: Discovering Your Conflict Management Style.
What is your natural take on conflict? Does even the word *conflict* strike fear into your heart?
Why or why not?

_____

_____

_____

When you lead others, will your fear of conflict be helpful or harmful? Why?

_____

_____

_____

Do you believe in a win-win approach to conflict management?

_____

Do you believe you can get past your fear to lead others toward a win-win? What are some ways
that you have successfully and previously used to manage fear in your life? Can you apply some of
these principles and strategies to when you need to manage conflict in the future?

_____

_____

_____

Anger

On the positive side, anger is basically an alert. It tells individuals that something may need to
be different in specific situations. Anger may notify individuals that they are ignoring an important
emotional issue or that their beliefs, values, passions, or needs are being compromised in some way.[9]
As an innate emotion, anger is connected to particular feelings, distinct thoughts, certain biological
and psychological states, and a range of behaviors.[10] Yet, anger may be difficult to understand, manage, or transform because people experience and express it in different ways and for different reasons. Something that makes one person furious may only mildly irritate someone else. For example,
while some people may verbalize mild unhappiness when someone cuts them off while driving in
traffic, others may become so angry that they shout loudly, swear, and then start driving aggressively
themselves. Ongoing changes in documentation requirements needed for prompt payment in health
care have caused physical therapist practice owners, managers, and clinicians to become angry about
doing more work for less payment.

Ultimately, individual responses to anger are controllable. One of the first steps for learning to
lead through conflict when there is anger is to become more aware of how to identify, express, and
manage anger, and then how to lead through the anger generated by others.

Box 8-1

DISCOVERING SOURCES OF ANGER

Following are some potential questions to ask to gain clarity around sources of anger:

- What am I really angry about?
- What is the problem, and whose problem is it?
- How can I sort out who is responsible for what?
- How can I learn to express my anger in a way that will not leave me feeling helpless and powerless?
- When I am angry, how can I clearly communicate my position without becoming defensive or attacking?
- What risks and losses might I face if I become clearer and more assertive?
- If getting angry is not working for me, what can I do differently?

Reprinted with permission from Lerner H. *The Dance of Anger.* New York, NY: Harper Collins Publishers; 1997:4.

A-HA! – WHAT MAKES YOU ANGRY?

Write down and reflect upon the times, people, and situations that make you angry.

_____

_____

_____

Ask yourself a few reflective questions to help you become more self-aware about your feelings of anger using the questions listed in Box 8-1: Discovering Sources of Anger.[9]

_____

_____

_____

Activity 8-3: How Effective Are You at Managing Your Anger?

Take the free Mindtools survey, "How Good Is Your Anger Management?" available at https://www.mindtools.com/pages/article/newTCS_88.htm.[11] Choose the response that best describes you. Answer the questions for how you are rather than how you think you should be.

Strategies to minimize situations that provoke frustration, stress, and anger, as well as those to reduce the effects of anger, are more easily recognized once self-assessment has occurred. Simple strategies may include changing the environment, understanding your triggers, using humor, and practicing relaxation techniques. More in-depth and longer-term strategies for anger management—including making improvements in communication, assertiveness, and team building—ironically fall within many of the same skills already discussed in this book. The goal in managing anger is to influence, direct, and redirect it so that it does not dominate emotions or actions or damage an important relationship or situation.

A-HA! – ANGER MANAGEMENT PLAN

Review your self-assessments in Box 8-1 and from the survey in Activity 8-3, then answer the following questions.

What are 3 things I can do to prevent or minimize anger in my life?

_____

_____

_____

What are 3 things I can do to productively redirect my anger when it occurs?

_____

_____

_____

How do others perceive my ability to control my anger and to help redirect the anger that others may express? (*Hint*: Ask for feedback on this one.)

_____

_____

_____

Microaggressions and Bullying

Microaggressions are described as short-lived, ordinary exchanges in which an individual directs straightforward condescending, arrogant, or demeaning verbal or nonverbal messages to certain individuals because of their group membership or other factors.[12] Name-calling, verbal attacks, and avoidant behavior are examples of microaggressions, referred to as *microassaults*, while subtle snubs or messages that convey rudeness and insensitivity are referred to as *microinsults*.[13] Unfortunately, microaggressions may be difficult to identify when they are occurring; usually individuals realize that the microaggressions have happened in retrospect. However, over time, the cumulative effect of microaggressions may lead to diminished trust within teams, decreased self-confidence of capable individuals, decreased satisfaction with work, and, ultimately, less-than-expected performance.

Individuals committing microaggressions may not intend to be offensive and may be unaware that they are causing harm.[12] Because microaggressions may be subtle, the recipients often dismiss a microaggressive experience, assume responsibility for it, or blame themselves for being overly sensitive. Perpetrators—if challenged—may defend their microaggressive behavior as a misunderstanding, a joke, or something small that was perhaps blown out of proportion.[12] However, microaggressions are a repeated approach to bullying and are exhibited frequently by individuals in peer-to-peer relationships and by people in positions or roles of authority or power. The harm inflicted by microaggressions may even be on par with overt bullying. This means that microaggressive behavior is formidable, significant, and perhaps even an unspoken threat that exists among individuals attempting to work together collaboratively in teams or organizations.

Unfortunately, *bullying* occurs within relationships as well as within the workplace, and bullying behavior worsens morale and productivity overall.[14] *Workplace bullying* is described as recurrent, health-damaging mistreatment of one or more persons by one or more perpetrators; it is driven

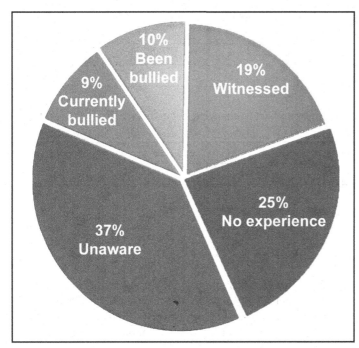

Figure 8-1. Prevalence of workplace bullying. (Adapted from Workplace Bullying Institute. *Workplace Bullying: US National Prevalence.* https://www.workplacebullying.org/2017-prevalence. Accessed March 27, 2020.)

by a perpetrators' need to control the targeted individual(s).[15] Workplace bullying is threatening, humiliating, or intimidating, and interferes or sabotages performance at work.[15] Bullying occurs in relationships in which the balance of power is somehow lopsided. Sadly, some leaders abuse their power simply because they can; they may be referred to as *bully bosses*. Bully bosses may use their power to hurt, demean, or take advantage of others who do not feel they are in a position to protect themselves. Regrettably, the prevalence of workplace bullying is staggering: 19% of workers are bullied, while an additional 19% witness it; Hispanics are the most frequently bullied race; 70% of the bullies are more likely to be men; 60% of the targets are women; women bullies target women in 67% of the cases; and 61% of Americans are aware now that workplace bullying happens (Figure 8-1).[15]

Preventing or limiting bullying, and covert relational aggressions, is a murky challenge, but one that needs to be addressed. Change requires leadership, and in the case of bullying, change requires courage, heightened awareness, and organizational factors to be reshaped explicitly.

Self-awareness is the starting point. For example, individuals may be experiencing bullying if their work or their contributions are never good enough; they feel caught off-guard when they are accused of incompetence despite a clear track record of top performance; they are called to surprise meetings everyone else knew about; and others on their team or at work have been told to stop working, talking, or socializing with them.[15]

After self-awareness, the next critical steps are to name the bullying or inappropriate behavior and identify viable options in which individuals can protect themselves, such as confront and/or report the inappropriate behavior, or line up another opportunity and leave the team or organization. Leading, especially during these difficult situations and within these conflicted relationships, takes moral courage (to be discussed further in Chapter 10 on ethics).

A-HA! – DANGEROUS BEHAVIORS

Have you ever been the target or witnesses of microaggressive behavior or bullying in the workplace?   Yes   No   I'm not sure

If so, did you do anything about it? Why or why not? Was your action effective?

_____

_____

_____

If not, do you feel you would know it now and act to change it if you did see it?

_____

_____

_____

•————————————

Apathy

The most common definitions for *apathy* include such things as absence of passion, emotion, or excitement; lack of interest or concern for matters of importance; and generalized indifference. This is nearly the opposite of the anger, microaggression, and bullying behaviors discussed previously, so it is difficult to imagine why apathy can be a barrier to conflict resolution, but it can be one of the biggest barriers a leader can face.

Recall from Chapter 6 the topic of engagement and its link to a team's effectiveness. Engagement expresses the active interest and desire to work toward the vision. In contrast, apathy of team members will be toxic to a team's performance, potentially infecting even the most engaged to become disengaged in the process. The same holds true in the teamwork required in conflict resolution. At least 2 parties are involved, and the vision for win-win will require the collaborative effort of each party. Some of the most difficult conflicts to manage are those involving disengaged, noncommunicative behaviors that stall and derail effective resolution. Reviewing the tips in Chapter 6 for engaging team members can help leaders learning to lead recognize and act to implement strategies to combat apathy with individual team members, although apathy can also be a product of a leader's lack of speed in addressing conflict or of a prolonged conflict situation.

People may become discouraged in a long-term conflict situation when there seems to be no possibility for change or a slim chance of ever being fully heard or understood. Each phase in a long-term conflict situation may be challenging, and it may seem easier just to avoid it. Continuing to stay engaged in the midst of ongoing conflict requires courage, skill, stamina, commitment, and support. Leaders should assure those involved that the matter is of importance and that steps are being made to find resolution. Leaders then need to maintain a consistent communication and dialogue with those involved in the conflict and move toward resolution with transparency of intent for a collaborative effort. In cases of unavoidably prolonged conflict, leaders may become more tolerant by using further strategies, such as the following:

- See the long-term. Accept that these issues, to some degree, may be with this group of individuals for some time. Do not let the conflict become all-consuming.
- Continue to relate to those with whom they are having difficulties.
- Look for opportunities to open a dialogue. Continue to affirm or acknowledge what matters to them and to understand how others see and feel about the issue(s).
- Celebrate small changes and positive interactions.
- Learn to recover from difficult interactions. Ask for help to understand what happened. Consider how these interactions might be contributing to the difficult interchange.
- Identify support resources and seek help, advice, and coaching.

A-HA! – LEADING THROUGH APATHY

Have you ever been involved in a team situation where certain members were not interested or not as passionate as you about the work involved?   Yes   No

How difficult was it for you to be around that team member? Did it create conflict within the group?

_____

_____

_____

Looking back, how could you use leadership skills to improve the situation and help re-engage that individual?

_____

_____

_____

Bottom Line!

Fear, anger, microaggression, bullying, and apathy all create conflict and impede effective resolution. Skilled leaders are able to recognize, name, and address these aversive behaviors toward facilitating mutual respect, although it requires significant awareness and moral courage. It may not be possible to avoid the dangers inherent to conflict, but it is possible to lead through them.

STRATEGIES IN LEADING THROUGH CONFLICT

Communicating, orchestrating, and negotiating are 3 strategies for leading yourself and others through conflict. As you read through this section, think about when and how each could be used most effectively in varied conflict situations.

Communicating

Conflict resolution does not occur without some form of communication taking place. Chapter 5 detailed the vast majority of the skills you will need to get started, including being aware of your communication styles as a leader and that of other parties, practicing vital listening skills, and effectively telling your story so others can understand. Two other strategies of further assistance in learning to lead through conflict are using the word "no," and employing nonviolent and compassionate communication techniques.

The Power of No

Believe it or not, saying "no" instead of giving in or compromising in a conflict, may lead to more creative and satisfying results for both parties. For example, S. Covey described the sixth paradigm of human interaction as win-win or no deal.[7] "No deal" is described as a situation in which a solution that benefits both parties (win-win) cannot be found, so the 2 parties agree to disagree agreeably.[7(p213)] At the start of the encounter, both parties state they want to go for win-win, but that if it comes to anything other than both parties getting what they desired, then they will both understand that an agreement will not be reached. This situation may occur when values or goals are simply not going in the same direction. If people enter the conversation with no deal as an option or as a possible outcome, then they are generally more open to try to really understand the deeper issues underlying viewpoints because they can always walk away.[7] Being able to fully collaborate on a potential solution, but then say, "No, this doesn't fit what I need," puts both parties at ease and makes them more likely to work together more fully from the start.

Remember that if everyone agreed on everything, then conflict would not exist. People disagree in conflict, which means that one party thinks "yes" and the other thinks "no." Collaboration (win-win) relies on both parties trusting each other to be honest so that each party can get what is desired from the engagement. If one individual does not have the capacity or the assertiveness skills to be able to say, "No, that won't solve our problem," then that person will most likely not benefit fully or at all with the outcome.

A-HA! – SAYING "NO"

Can you remember a time, possibly in a team situation, when you wanted to say, "No," but you wound up agreeing either just to end the conflict, even though the result did not meet your needs?
Yes   No

What held you back from saying "No"?

_____

_____

_____

As a leader, do you feel you would be able to invite others to speak their minds even if you knew it would prolong a resolution?

_____

_____

_____

●————————————

Nonviolent and Compassionate Communication

Nonviolent communication, or compassionate communication, is one way for leaders to mediate disputes and conflicts at all levels. It is founded on language and communication skills that strengthen a leader's ability to remain calm, even under trying conditions.[16] This approach guides leaders to reframe how they express themselves precisely, and to listen to others by focusing their consciousness on the 4 areas of observing, feeling, need, and request, as shown in Figure 8-2 and detailed next[17]:

- Observing: Individuals observe what is happening in a situation. For example, they observe what others are doing or saying. The key is to express this observation simply and without introducing any judgment or evaluation.
  - "I noticed that it was 8:15 am when you arrived; the meeting was scheduled to begin at 7:45 am."
- Feeling: Individuals state clearly and honestly how they feel when they observe this action. For example, they tell others if they are scared, hurt, happy, amused, or irritated.
  - "I felt irritated at first that you were late, and then I got concerned that something might have happened to prevent you from making it to the meeting at the time it was scheduled."

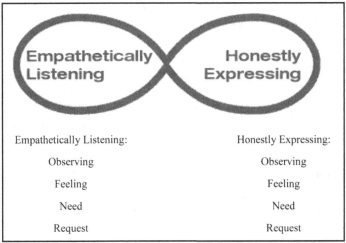

Figure 8-2. The nonviolent communication process. (Reprinted with permission from The Nonviolent Communication Model, The Center for Nonviolent Communication, Albuquerque, NM. Available at https://www.cnvc.org/Training/the-nvc-model. Accessed February 3, 2018.)

- Need: Individuals state their needs in connection with their identified feelings.
  - "I need full participation from all team members to make these meeting productive."
- Request: Individuals make a request.
  - "I want to make sure that we use our meeting time and our energy as productively as possible. I know that we are all busy. Therefore, it is critical for us to start and stop our meetings on time. As a member of this team, I am asking that you to arrive on time, every time."

Nonviolent communication trains leaders learning to lead to reveal behaviors and conditions that are affecting them through an approach that fosters deep listening, respect, and empathy. Leaders also learn how to identify and articulate their needs in a given situation. This approach is simple, yet may be powerfully transformative. Through this approach, leaders may start to perceive old patterns of behavior, themselves, others, their intentions, and relationships in a new light. To learn more about nonviolent communication training, visit the Center for Nonviolent Communication website at www.cnvc.org or get resources at www.nonviolentcommunication.com.[17]

Orchestrating

Orchestrating conflict is described as designing and leading the process of change by getting participants to work through their differences productively.[18] In this section, 2 models are discussed: adaptive leadership[18] and dialogue principles for crucial conversations.[4]

Adaptive Leadership

In his book, *Leadership Without Easy Answers*, Heifetz describes *adaptive leadership* as a set of strategies and practices used by leaders to break through deadlocks, accomplish deep change, and develop the adaptability to succeed in complex, competitive, and challenging environments.[19] Essentially, leadership that is adaptive is about leading change needed to enable teams, organizations, and systems to thrive. Adaptive leaders and leaders learning to lead can use 7 steps to start this process of orchestrating conflict.[18] It is a good idea to introduce these specific steps to the entire group at the beginning so that everyone is clear about the process that will be used to tackle the conflict. These 7 steps are as follows[18]:

1. Prepare: Before surfacing any conflict intentionally, thoroughly seek and review information such as the history and background leading up to the current problem or issue; the people involved in the situation, either directly or indirectly; any strategies the group has already attempted to use; any progress the group has been able to make so far; and any barriers encountered.

2. Establish ground rules: Establish common rules of engagement up front to create a safe place for confidential discussions. An example of a ground rule is to speak directly to each other to seek clarification about intent or specific content to enhance understanding.

3. Facilitate the discussion in such a way to get each and every view on the table: Specify and clarify the issues of both or all sides. This step requires courage, openness, and honesty from all team members.

4. Orchestrate the conflict: It is the leader's role as the facilitator to explicitly state all of the competing issues and positions, and then to restate and possibly reframe the big picture or the work that the entire group needs to do. For example, the leader can identify that subgroup A supports X while subgroup B supports Y, and that the group still needs to do W. In this way, the leader may start to uncover areas of common ground or shared interest.

5. Encourage accepting and managing losses: Both subgroups may have to give up some things to achieve W. Take time to identify and reflect on possible losses that may be experienced as a result of new alternatives or new pathways being suggested. This step may help others let go of their losses—real or perceived—and move forward.

6. Allow for people to experiment: Make a shared commitment to determine how to tackle the challenges and how to implement new courses of action. Allow time to evaluate and modify strategies as needed over a certain period of time.

7. Encourage peers to consult with each other to maximize the chances of success: Allow time and space for members of the group to consult informally with each other about the merits and anticipated challenges of the new action plan.

Adaptive leadership is needed for conflicts or problems that are adaptive in nature, such as the problems and conflicts related to fixing the US health care system. Health care reform is not a quick fix; rather, it is a problem that is intricate and involves the highly varied opinions and visions of many sectors. There are many smaller-based adaptive challenges faced every day, and the 7 steps for orchestrating conflict guide the adaptive leader to seek out others' interpretations about the conflict to see things from a different viewpoint for a more comprehensive, collaborative pool of solutions.

Conversations That Are Critical

A second useful model for orchestrating conflict can be found in the 7 dialogue principles detailed in the book *Crucial Conversations*, in which a *crucial conversation* is defined as "a discussion between 2 or more people where stakes are high, opinions vary, and emotions run strong."[4(p3)] These could be the conversations needed when you believe you deserve a raise but your supervisor does not, or when you feel like the performance of a colleague is not in the best interest of the patient and something needs to be said. Basically, the need for crucial conversations most likely happens every day, but, like most conflict, may not get addressed to resolution or at all.

Facing these conflict situations can be challenging, although it can be faced effectively using the skills of the 7 dialogue principles[4]:

1. Start with the heart: Determining what you really want for you, others, and the relationship

2. Learn to look: Remaining alert for when the conversation may be getting crucial to the point of safety issues for you or the other party, and looking to ensure you stay calm under stress

3. Make it safe: Taking action to re-establish the safety of both parties by apologizing when appropriate, using contrast to fix a misunderstanding, and re-establishing mutual respect and purpose

4. Master your stories: Determining what story you have told yourself to get to this point in the conflict, and considering the rest of the story that may be different now that you know more about the other person's position

5. State your path: Sharing the facts, telling your story, asking for others' paths, talking tentatively, and encouraging testing of the issues and potential solutions

6. Explore others' paths: Ensuring empathy by asking, mirroring, paraphrasing, reframing, and priming to actively explore others' views by agreeing, building, and comparing on their views

7. Move to action: Assisting the conversation toward deciding how a decision will be made, and following through to ensure solutions are implemented in that way

A-HA! – YOUR LAST CRITICAL CONVERSATION

Think of the last high-stakes, opposing-opinion, or strong-emotion conversation that you had. What was it about?

_____

_____

_____

How did you handle it?

_____

_____

_____

How did your actions compare to the 7 dialogue principles listed above?

_____

_____

_____

If you had to do it all over again, what would you change? Why would this change have made a difference?

_____

_____

_____

The model using the 7 dialogue principles for crucial conversations, like any other process, requires training and deliberate practice. These skills are definitely worth learning, as conflict situations often require these types of conversations. Further information regarding training in this method is available at www.vitalsmarts.com/crucial-conversations-training.

Negotiating

Negotiating involves discussing, debating, and reaching a mutually satisfactory agreement. It has been discussed throughout this entire chapter. Many conflicts can be resolved, without thinking of them as a formal negotiation process, by using some of the models and strategies already mentioned including trusting, empathizing, effectively communicating needs and intentions, and orchestrating conflict. Ury describes negotiation as a back-and-forth process of communication aimed at reaching agreement with others in which some interests are shared while others are opposed.[5] He also adds that "negotiation is not limited to the activity of formally sitting across a table discussing a contentious issue; it is the informal activity you engage in whenever you try to get something you want from another person."[5(p4)] All of the skills learned in this chapter, and those leading up to this chapter, already strengthen a leader's capacity for effectiveness in negotiation.

Box 8-2

NEGOTIATION TIPS

- Plan in advance for your conversation.
  - Decide on your main concerns on the issue, and brainstorm what you believe to be key concerns that the other side may have.
  - Understand the common ground between both parties, focusing on the problem and not the people.
  - Create a list of options for discussion once the conversation begins, and be prepared to be flexible.
  - Know your bottom line, and prepare yourself to walk away if a joint agreement cannot be established.
- Meet to negotiate (face-to-face is the best when possible).
  - State the concern that you have on this matter and the importance that this issue represents for you.
  - Ask the other person to share concerns on this matter.
  - Adjust your previously brainstormed list of options based on both your perspective and the other person's verified concerns.
  - Understand any forces outside your control that may be affecting the problem, and adjust your strategy accordingly.
  - Offer potential options for agreement on the matter, and listen to options of the other party.
  - Decide on a course of action, and come to an agreement, if possible. If there is no potential for acceptable agreement, be ready to walk away rather than concede to something you do not want to agree to. It is difficult to do, but sometimes necessary.
  - Summarize the conversation and outcome. Get details of any agreement reached in writing.

Activity 8-4: Improving Your Negotiation Skills

Consider the practices detailed in Box 8-2. Reflect on the lessons in this chapter to determine in which of the following negotiation skills you could use the most improvement. List 3 areas that you will focus on in your next conflict negotiation.

1. _____
2. _____
3. _____

Leaders Helping Leaders: A Third Party

Even the best leaders, conflict orchestrators, and negotiators can use help sometimes. This could mean simply having someone to talk to, off-the-record, who is not directly or indirectly involved in the conflict. This objective person may offer some coaching, support, empathy, or suggestions on how to approach the conflict better or differently. Conflict may need to be handled in this way in organizations because no other formal systems are established to deal with conflict, except for those conflicts stemming from poor performance. For intragroup conflicts, organizations may hold a specific forum, mediated by an objective party, in which each group is invited to express concerns openly. Using a mediator to manage conflict may help to facilitate a more productive dialogue. These forums may also provide an opportunity for groups to brainstorm about what to do next, or how to come to acceptance with the outcome of the conflict.

Finally, when an entrenched conflict exists (ie, when the behaviors associated with the conflict become more comfortable than potential change) no one may be motivated to make any change. Therefore, third-party assistance may be helpful in these situations by mapping out the effects and the cost of the longstanding conflict and by helping people see how the conflict affects all other aspects of their work and daily lives. This third party may be able to provide options about how to make even small adjustments to start chipping away at the ineffective patterns of interacting.

Bottom Line!

"Anyone can hold the helm when the sea is calm." – Publilius Syrus, Latin writer

With the right skills and practice, those learning to lead can hold the helm at all times.

Case Study: Using Conflict to Initiate Change

It was obvious to Jamie, as the new center manager, that the clinic needed to make changes immediately to achieve senior management's performance expectations. However, clinical team members appeared comfortable with how things had been working under the former center manager. The members of this team made it clear to Jamie that they were eager to preserve the status quo to maintain their current level of performance. When Jamie started in her new role, the physical therapy clinic was open Mondays through Fridays from 9 am until 5 pm. However, Jamie discovered quickly that many of the current (and potential) patients/clients, commuted every day to work, either downtown to the major metropolitan area or to the neighboring suburbs. This meant that their patient population started their commute to work early in the morning and did not return to the area until later in the evening. Jamie sensed quickly that the clinic was limiting its own daily performance and access to its potential client/patient population as a direct result of these limited hours of operation. She knew that the operating hours had to expand, but she also knew this change would create conflict and resistance within her team.

Jamie called a team meeting specifically to discuss the changes that needed to be made to the clinic's hours of operation. As she prepared for the meeting, she considered using 2 approaches:

1. Approach 1: Jamie thought that it might be valuable to tell her team that the senior management team perceived the clinic to be underperforming, overstaffed, and losing patients to the competition due to its inflexible schedule. In this way, Jamie believed she would get immediate buy-in from the team because "management said so" as she announced the plan to expand their clinic hours from 7 am until 7:30 pm, Monday through Friday, effective immediately, and to add Saturday hours within 2 months.

2. Approach 2: Jamie thought that having an open dialogue as a group about the need to expand the hours of the clinic would be the best way to introduce the changes that had to occur. She knew that changing the schedule would create conflict, but she knew that she could not avoid this conflict any longer.

After careful preparation, Jamie decided it was her responsibility to initiate and lead the change process. She did not want to use senior management's perceptions as the only reasons why the schedule needed to change. She knew that she had to explain what needed to change and why based on her own observations and conclusions, not based on senior management's directives. By assuming responsibility for this management decision, Jamie felt she would continue to build credibility within her own team, despite the conflict. Jamie decided to orchestrate the change process proactively by using the 7 steps as identified by Heifet (Table 8-2).

Chapter Key Words

Conflict, Trust, Empathy, Assertiveness, Cooperativeness, Microaggression, Bullying, Adaptive Leadership, Negotiating

References

1. Cambridge English Dictionary. *Conflict.* http://dictionary.cambridge.org/us/dictionary/english/conflict. Accessed October 30, 2018.

2. Mayer Bernard. *Staying With Conflict: A Strategic Approach to Ongoing Disputes.* Hoboken, NJ: John Wiley & Sons; 2009.

3. Covey SMR. *The SPEED of TRUST: The One Thing That Changes Everything.* New York, NY: Simon & Schuster; 2006.

4. Patterson K, Grenny J, McMillan R, Switzler A. *Crucial Conversations: Tools for Talking When Stakes Are High.* Updated second edition. Singapore: McGraw-Hill Education; 2012.

5. Ury W. *Getting Past No: Negotiating Your Way from Confrontation to Cooperation.* Rev ed. New York, NY: Bantam Books; 1993.

6. *Thomas-Kilmann Conflict Mode Instrument (TKI).* http://www.cpp.com/en-US/Products-and-Services/TKI. Accessed October 10, 2018.

7. Covey SR. *The 7 Habits of Highly Effective People: Restoring the Character Ethic.* First Fireside edition. New York,NY: Fireside Book; 1990.

8. Lencioni P. *The Five Dysfunctions of a Team: A Leadership Fable.* 1st ed. San Francisco, CA: Jossey-Bass; 2002. http://www.books24x7.com/marc.asp?bookid=3740. Accessed October 10, 2018.

9. Lerner HG. *The Dance of Anger: A Woman's Guide to Changing the Patterns of Intimate Relationships.* 1st William Morrow paperback edition. New York, NY: William Morrow & Co, an imprint of HarperCollins Publishers; 2014.

10. Goleman D. *Emotional Intelligence: Why It Can Matter More than IQ.* London, UK: Bloomsbury; 1996.

11. Mindtools. *How Good is Your Anger Management?* https://www.mindtools.com/pages/article/newTCS_88.htm. Accessed April 18, 2019.

12. Sue DW. *Microaggressions and Marginality: Manifestation, Dynamics, and Impact.* Hoboken, NJ: John Wiley & Sons; 2010.

13. Sue DW. *Microaggressions in Everyday Life: Race, Gender, and Sexual Orientation.* Hoboken, NJ: John Wiley & Sons; 2010.

14. Sutton RI. *The No Asshole Rule: Building a Civilized Workplace and Surviving One That Isn't.* New York, NY: Business Plus; 2010.

15. Workplace Bullying Institute. *Workplace Bullying: US National Prevalence.* https://www.workplacebullying.org/2017-prevalence. Accessed March 27, 2020.

16. Rosenberg MB. *Speak Peace in a World of Conflict: What You Say Next Will Change Your World.* Encinitas, CA: Puddle Dancer Press; 2005.

TABLE 8-2. JAMIE'S APPROACH TO ORCHESTRATING CONFLICT	
STEP 1	Before taking any action, Jamie considered 2 ways to approach the conversation with her team, and considered the pros and cons of each approach. She decided to approach her team using more of participative leadership style (approach 2) vs an authoritarian (telling) style (approach 1). Jamie learned more about her own conflict management style (gained self-awareness by completing the TKI Conflict Mode self-assessment) so she could lead through this conflict better. She decided to try to use a collaborative or win-win conflict management style. This decision meant that Jamie needed to be more assertive in communicating why the changes needed to occur, and to be more cooperative in working with her team to design the new schedule. Jamie considered how each person on her team would react to the schedule changes by trying to anticipate each person's conflict management styles.
STEP 2	During the team meeting, Jamie explained the changes they needed to make (what), why they needed to make the changes, and then outlined a suggested process they could use to design the new schedule (how). They established a few ground rules in advance to help them proactively identify how they would make their final decisions. Example of a ground rule: Everyone must participate in providing input in designing the new schedule.
STEP 3	Jamie asked each member of her team to provide input regarding their preferences (ie, ideal schedule), any restrictions they had (ie, evening[s] they could not work because of night classes), and any pending vacations/time off. Jamie gave her team members 1 week to provide input. She compiled all the input into one spreadsheet and shared the information with everyone for review. Jamie had to follow up with the office coordinator directly when she did not provide her input. At the second team meeting, they reviewed the input and brainstormed together how they could create a schedule that was fair for everyone.
STEP 4	In the second team meeting, Jamie highlighted the clinic hours that were covered and those that were not covered. She proposed 2 ways in which they could redesign the schedule so that all hours were covered, and asked the team for input/other ideas.
STEP 5	Jamie gave her team members 1 week between meetings to get used to the decision to change the schedule, and allowed each person to provide input individually before discussing the new schedule as a group.
STEP 6	Jamie suggested that they try the new schedule for 1 month as a pilot, and then regroup as a team to discuss what was working and what was not working, and to change it for the second month as needed.
STEP 7	This opportunity was built into the change process by allowing time between discussions for peers to talk with each other, and by implementing the new schedule as a pilot.

17. Center for Nonviolent Communication: A Global Organization. https://www.cnvc.org/index. Accessed October 10, 2018.

18. Heifetz RA, Grashow A, Linsky M. *The Practice of Adaptive Leadership: Tools and Tactics for Changing Your Organization and the World*. Cambridge, MA: Harvard Business Press; 2009.

19. Heifetz RA. *Leadership Without Easy Answers*. Vol 465. Cambridge, MA: Harvard University Press; 1994.

SUGGESTED READINGS

Fisher R, Ury W, Patton B. *Getting to Yes: Negotiating Agreement Without Giving In*. New York, NY: Penguin Books; 2011.

Patterson K, Grenny J, McMillan R, Switzler A. *Crucial Conversations: Tools for Talking When Stakes Are High*. New York, NY: McGraw-Hill; 2012.

Ury W. *Getting Past No: Negotiating in Difficult Situations*. New York, NY: Bantam Books; 1993:171.

UNIT 3

LEADERSHIP AND CHANGE
WHY IT MATTERS

Change is inevitable, especially in health care. Change is needed for many reasons, and there are benefits to be gained from change. Individuals and organizations change over time to adapt to external pressures, improve performance, build capabilities, strengthen behavior, and enhance outcomes. Change requires leadership, and recall that in this book, leadership is about action and behavior.

In Unit 1, you discovered the first person that you lead is you! The term *personal leadership* described self-leadership or this act of leading from inside out. It is a self-driven style in which you are the facilitator of your own life. Developing effective personal leadership skills starts with personal change.

In Unit 2, emphasis was on exploring how you can lead as a collaborative member of any group, and how some leadership styles are more effective than others, especially at engaging and inspiring teams to action. Developing better relationships, collaboration, and teamwork requires *all* individuals within a team to change and adapt their own individual behaviors, and as a result, they will transform how they work together.

This unit examines the leadership skills needed to inspire and influence forward-looking change within different contexts, and why change matters.

Leading Change

Jennifer Green-Wilson, PT, MBA, EdD

What good is an idea if it remains an idea?
Try. Experiment. Iterate. Fail. Try again. Change the world.

— *Simon Sinek, author of* Start With Why:
How Great Leaders Inspire Everyone to Take Action

CHAPTER OBJECTIVES

- › Discuss why change requires leadership skills.
- › Self-assess your approach to change.
- › Identify benefits of change.
- › Discuss types of change.
- › Examine change as a process.
- › Discuss how you can build readiness for change.
- › Identify one way in which you can lead change proactively.

Green-Wilson J, Zeigler S, eds.
Learning to Lead in Physical Therapy (pp 159-174).
© 2020 Taylor & Francis Group.

Leadership Vignette

Diane E. Clark, PT, DScPT, MBA

Leading change requires time, energy, and an intentional approach. This approach worked well when we introduced interprofessional simulation into the doctor of physical therapy curriculum. Faculty members understood the why behind making this important change. We all understood that we needed training to do it well. As the role model leading this new approach to teaching and learning, I shared a roadmap for others to go about becoming trained. We explored existing on-campus events and developed relationships with other professional programs in the School of Health Professions to incorporate interprofessional learning activities into the curriculum. I became trained and worked with people on campus to develop our first simulation. Then, I invited others to join in, and had an early follower who later became an expert. Others followed and joined the "dance" ("First Follower: Leadership Lessons from the Dancing Guy," available at https://www.youtube. com/watch?v=fW8amMCVAJQ). People bought into the concepts because they could see the benefits to the students in learning in this newer format. Ultimately, we knew we had been successful in leading this change when our students provided very positive feedback! The faculty members continue to work on integrating more opportunities that are both formative and summative into the curriculum, and disseminating our success.

Other times, leading change was more challenging. Focus groups with clinical instructors, site coordinators of clinical education, and employers revealed that competencies, which would later be identified as personal leadership, were needed if our graduates were to be successful in the dynamic health care environment. As early adopters of incorporating Personal Leadership (PL) as a curricular thread into the doctor of physical therapy curriculum, the faculty members struggled to find a common voice. As we struggled to define this change process, my role was to be cheerleader and champion of the cause, continually reminding everyone of the why behind the change. Even though we were intentional about making this change, we initially did not invest enough upfront time to gain a collective buy-in or develop our shared vision together. Upon reflection, I realized several aspects made leading this change more difficult. Although faculty members bought into the fact that PL was important for the success of our graduates, both faculty and students felt that they knew what personal leadership was and what competencies related to PL. As we attempted to incorporate PL as a curricular thread, we were all over the map—in our use of language related to PL, and in what we identified as the necessary competencies. Trying to get consensus led to conflict and resistance to change. We determined that we needed an explicit intervention to keep us moving forward. Consequently, we invested in and required all faculty to participate in LAMP 101, a weekend course on personal leadership, to standardize our language and our approach to developing PL competencies in the curriculum. We also involved clinicians and employers from the community in the change process, and continued to ensure that their voices were heard as stakeholders in the educational process. Our clinical faculty and employers of graduates are essential members of our educational team, and their role as champions of PL was critical to establishing its street credibility with our students. In hindsight, I wish we had spent more time early on exploring faculty members' readiness for this change, and assessing beliefs, values, and knowledge related to PL. I believe that taking time to build this foundation would have enabled us as a faculty to move ahead sooner and implement this curricular thread more seamlessly.

We all know that change is difficult because it requires behaviors to change. As faculty members, we tend to relate leading as what we do with our patients and clients, and changing behaviors as a goal we engage in with them. Most of us [faculty members] view ourselves as having individual mandates related to teaching, scholarship, and service, and not as being influential members of the department team. Change moves people out of comfort zones and may require the work of reflection and self-assessment to perhaps learn skills and knowledge unrelated to our core expertise—the soft skills that need to be employed in a different content and role modeled for students. Given busy workloads, we all fall back on what is easier (less work). However, faculty members are tasked with leading and responding to change that is occurring in health care so that our graduates are successful as change agents in meeting the evolving needs of health care consumers and the health care market. While our mission and vision may remain the same, how we go about getting to that mission and vision must change in order for educational programs to remain relevant and transform society. To transform society, we, as educators and role models for future generations of physical therapists and health care professionals, need to transform ourselves in all aspects of education, service, practice, and research.

Leading change is not easy; expect resistance, and spend enough time throughout the process to build the foundations for success. You cannot overstate the why or the need for change. Framing the right context for change is important; otherwise, it becomes change for change's sake. If you ascribe to the fundamental belief that faculty, students, and graduates want to be doing the best job and striving for excellence, then approach them from this perspective. As a leader, build your growth mindset and remember that your attitude and energy toward leading change is everything! Engage others in the process early on to get buy-in and to share ideas. Provide the tools and resources needed for success, and hold everyone accountable for making the change happen. Celebrate milestones achieved along the way! Have those difficult conversations with individuals who are actively or passively sabotaging the team's efforts so that team energy can be focused on achieving the goal.

I strongly believe we need to keep changing intentionally within physical therapy. Doing the same thing as we did 10 or even 5 years ago will not allow us to meet our new vision for our profession. Given student debt load and flat salaries, current educational models are not sustainable. Having tunnel vision—that the only person who is important is the patient in front of you—will not allow physical therapy as a profession to thrive and be seen as a solution to the problem of health care financing and mediocre outcomes. Physical therapists must effectively lead themselves and others in daily practice and be seen as valuable and effective team members advocating for the individual patient, and also collectively for society. Blinders need to come off, and we need to be involved at the organizational, community, and national levels. We offer answers to many issues prevalent today, and we need to be proud of our skill sets, scope of practice, and ability to lead change across all settings and industries.

We have an opportunity to lead transformational change. *Transformational change* has been around since 1973, when the term was coined by James V. Downton. In 1978, leadership expert James Burns defined *transformational leadership* as a process "where leaders and their followers raise one another to higher levels of morality and motivation."[7(p 20)] Transformational change is a fundamental process needed today for physical therapy educators and clinicians to respond to the rapid, dynamic marketplace of health care. We no longer have the luxury to take 5 years to implement a curricular change or address practice processes and outcomes. We need to be nimble, be connected to our external stakeholders, and leverage our political savvy to advocate and lobby for our profession. The strategies, processes, and leadership of transformational change need to become intrinsic values of the culture of institutions and practices. Imagine our future when education and practice within physical therapy both meet and anticipate the needs of the individual, community, organization, and profession. What if we embrace change and dare to lead? The *what if* has now become the next vital sign for our profession to succeed, and benchmarks for our survival. Our call to action is now, and leading transformational change is our bridge to the future.

CHANGE REQUIRES LEADERSHIP

Leadership influences change, and change is a fundamental domain of leadership.[1] Leaders are forward-looking and tend to be restless with the status quo. Leaders are positive and optimistic about the future, and they passionately believe they can make a difference.[1] Leaders seek out and accept challenging opportunities to stretch their own abilities and the capacity of others.

Inspired leaders think, act, and communicate from the inside out.[2] They motivate others toward change by communicating the why behind the change—the reason for it, why people should care about it, and why it will make a difference.[2] Through displaying their energy and optimism, leaders inspire people to initiate change, take on risk, do things differently, and make things happen.

A-HA! – YOU AND CHANGE

Identify a time you had to change something, such as how you changed your approach to your work, your hobbies, or your daily routine.

What was easy about making this change? Why?

_____

_____

_____

What was difficult about making this change? Why?

_____

_____

_____

When you made this change, did it make things easier or better? Why?

_____

_____

_____

BENEFITS OF CHANGE

Opportunities change, technologies change, and over time, people change. Recall the last time you changed something. Did you make this change because you wanted to make it or because you had to make it? Change can refer to the process used to cause a task, practice, or activity to become different in some way compared to what it is at the present or what it was in the past. For example, an organization or department can change its process of hiring physical therapists. Change can also describe the effects or outcomes after an activity, task, or method has transformed. For example, physical therapists may find it easier to practice on a daily basis after they simplify their master scheduling system.

People do not like to change much, yet change is inevitable—especially in health care.

People prefer to maintain the status quo. They like to avoid rocking the boat and remain in their comfort zone; therefore, they tend to avoid change whenever they can. Still, change is needed for many reasons, and there are benefits to be gained from change. A few of these benefits include opportunity, flexibility, experience, confidence, personal growth, improvement, and resilience. As you read the next few sections, think about which benefits are most important for you in terms of leading change.

Opportunity

Imagine your lifestyle if you did the exact same thing at the exact same time in the exact same way every day. Even though this approach to living may seem comfortable because it is predictable, it can also be rather uninteresting and monotonous. Learning to embrace change can expand your opportunities in many ways. In addition to personal and professional growth, new opportunities resulting from change may bring you novel experiences that could open you to new sources of energy, excitement, and satisfaction.

A-HA! – SEEKING OPPORTUNITIES FOR CHANGE

How often do you change your daily routine? Why or why not?

_____
_____
_____

Do you seek new opportunities? How do you do this, and how often?

_____
_____
_____

What motivates you to pursue something new?

_____
_____
_____

Flexibility

The shifting dynamics within health care mean that you will need to adapt and respond to change quickly. Most likely, the health care team will consider you an asset if you learn to adapt well to shifting priorities. Furthermore, experiencing change helps you learn to be more flexible, more agile, and possibly more open-minded. Resisting change can lead to unnecessary stress. Therefore, being flexible will make you more responsive to change and will help you adapt to new situations, new environments, and new people more easily.

Activity 9-1: How Flexible and Adaptable Are You to Change?

Health care organizations are looking for team members who have adaptable mindsets and can be flexible. The good news is that you can develop and improve your skills to be flexible and adaptable to change. Do you know how adaptable you are, and does it change in different situations? Read the 2 scenarios below, and select one choice that best captures your typical response. Afterward, think about what you need to do to be more flexible or adaptable. Why do you think this new approach would make a difference?

Scenario 1: To meet an increased demand for patient care, you have to work every Saturday for the next month. You think:

A. No way, my weekends are for me.

B. Yes, *but…* we obviously need to provide coverage for our patients, but I'll only do it if I'm paid extra for the hours that I work.

C. Of course! This is good news for the future of our health care organization! Sign me up! What shifts do you need covered?

D. I don't have a choice; I might get in trouble if I say no.

Your "typical" response (select 1):   A   B   C   D

Scenario 2: Your supervisor calls. Her car broke down 30 miles from your health system and she is stuck. She asks you to rearrange your schedule quickly so you can pick her up. You think:

A. I'm not an Uber service. She needs to figure it out.

B. Yes, of course! I'll leave as soon as I can.

C. I really don't prefer to do this, but I will because it's a professional obligation (ie, it's my duty to help my supervisor; she called *me* for help).

D. Before I say yes or no, let's brainstorm to see if you have any other options. I'm worried about taking care of my patients

Your "typical" response (select 1):   A   B   C   D

Experience

Change is hard, and it is often hard to make change happen. Yet, the best way to learn is through experience, and learning can occur from both positive and negative experiences. *Experience* is the process of gaining knowledge and skills from doing, seeing, or feeling different things. Experience refers to gaining a comprehensive understanding or know-how about something. For example, a physical therapist can gain a reputation as an expert clinician with considerable experience.

Confidence

Confidence is the feeling of self-assurance resulting from when you appreciate your own abilities or qualities. Individuals display self-confidence by attempting new things, being decisive and focused, and remaining in control during difficult situations. People with high self-confidence seem to exude enthusiasm and passion. Others tend to trust and respect passionate and confident individuals, which helps build even more self-confidence. You gain confidence, or a state of being certain, through experience, and you can gain confidence when you experience change. Change requires taking risks, and gaining confidence will fuel your capacity to take on risk and lead change.

Activity 9-2: How Self-Confident Are You?

In general, how self-confident are you? Are there times when you feel more confident than other times? Take the "How Confident Are You" self-assessment[3] found at https://www.mindtools.com/pages/article/newTCS_84.htm.

Review and reflect upon your results. Identify one situation in which your lack of self-confidence is holding you back to help determine a strategy or strategies to break through this barrier. Determine what help you might need, and what you would need to do differently.

Personal Growth

A key aspect of developing personal leadership skills is seeking opportunities for personal growth. You grow and learn new things every time something changes and, sometimes, you make changes intentionally to help you grow as an individual. *Personal growth*, or self-improvement, refers to when you guide your own development so that you realize your potential better. You change how you think and what you do so that you can leverage your strengths, passions, and capabilities in different ways. By doing so, you discover new insights about aspects of your life while interacting with others. You learn lessons even from the changes that did not lead you to where you thought you would end up or where you wanted to be. You can even learn great lessons from changes that resulted in failure. Discussions about leading personal change will continue throughout this chapter and the rest of this book.

A-HA! – PERSONAL CHANGE REFLECTION

Throughout this book, you have been encouraged to make personal changes. Take a few moments to reflect on your personal leadership development journey so far.

What changes have you already made? Why did you make these changes? What difference did they make? Why?

_____

_____

_____

What changes do you still want to make, and why have you not made these changes yet?

_____

_____

_____

Improvement

Think about the things that you would like to improve in your life—relationships, grades, personal finances, fitness/activity level, eating habits, and so on. You know that these opportunities most likely will not get better if you do not do something differently or explicitly to make them happen. Without change, no significant improvements would be made. Maintaining the status quo breeds mediocrity, whereas change triggers progress. Things move forward and develop because of change.

Resilience

Recall from Chapter 1 that *resilience*, or hardiness, describes a process of adapting well to change. It means being able to bounce back from change—perhaps from difficult experiences such as failure, adversity, or trauma.[4] Recall also that resilient people view difficulty, such as change, as a challenge, not as a paralyzing event, and that building resilience involves learning and developing specific behaviors, thoughts, and actions. For example, resilient people look at their failures and mistakes as lessons from which they can learn, and as opportunities for growth. Through self-reflection, individuals can learn something about themselves and may find that they have grown in some respect because of their struggle with loss or failure. They do not view failure as a negative reflection on their own abilities or self-worth. Developing resilience is a personal journey. One approach to building resilience that works for one person might not work for another because people do not react the same to traumatic or stressful life events.

A-HA! – HOW DO YOU SEE FAILURE?

Identify a situation or a change you made that you would describe as a failure. Why was it a failure from your perspective?

_____

_____

_____

How did you bounce back from this not-so-positive situation? What did you do? Or, if you did not yet bounce back fully, why not? Reflect upon what is holding you back.

_____

_____

_____

Upon reflection, what lessons did you learn from this failure? How does this experience inform you about facing future difficult situations?

_____

_____

_____

Bottom Line!

Ongoing reform, everchanging business models, innovations in technology, and other anticipated changes in health care will continue to impact physical therapist practice. Therefore, both organizations and people are demanding deep change with an increased frequency. Responsive organizations and health care professionals need to be open, courageous, and responsive to lead change.

TYPES OF CHANGE

Many types of change exist. Researchers describe change as planned, ongoing, radical, chaotic, or transformational. They identify underlying reasons why change occurs, and investigate failures as growth opportunities. Individuals change and organizations change, so change is required in response. Sometimes change is minor, and sometimes it is major and all-encompassing. Essentially, change is a constant, especially in health care. Change may develop from within a health care system, or because it needs to adopt or adapt to something new and imposed external to it.[5] External factors—which include economic uncertainties, health care reform, and changes in government regulations—play a crucial role in compelling health care systems and organizations to change. Because you will face change every day as a health care professional and you need to carry this task out successfully, it is essential to recognize the types of change that you may encounter. Being able to differentiate among these types of change will help you develop your leadership skills to lead through change effectively.

Health care anticipates change to be constant, and while proactive individuals and companies embrace this, not all change is planned nor predictable. *Planned change* occurs when deliberate decisions, planning, and goal-setting made by an individual or organization causes changes to happen, while *unplanned change* may result from unforeseen circumstances or lack of planning. Planned change describes a deliberate alteration in the status quo by means of a carefully formulated process. In 1947, Lewin developed a theory or model of planned change based on 3 successive stages or phases of change: unfreezing, moving or changing, and refreezing.[6] Lewin described unfreezing of the existing system of interests and relationships as the stage of liberating the individual/organization for possible change, moving the individual or organization to the new level of planned or desired behaviors or structures, and refreezing the new behaviors or systems as a sustainable integration of the changes made. He suggested that individuals or organizations had to become unfrozen to offset complacency, status quo, and stasis by displacing customary patterns and routines. Planned changes can be implemented by collaborative or coercive means, or through imitating others.

Incremental change is usually a result of logical analysis and planning. For example, an individual or a team could identify a desired goal with specific steps or changes that would have to be made to achieve it. Incremental change is usually limited in scope, often reversible, and does not disrupt performance patterns too much. If change made incrementally does not work out, teams could always return to the old way of doing things. Making incremental changes may help individuals feel as if they are still in control during the process of change. In contrast, *deep change* is more difficult, and it can occur at the organizational and personal levels. Deep change tends to be meaningful, significant in scope, multifaceted, and usually irreversible. Deep change differs from incremental change in that it requires new ways of thinking and behaving. The effort to make deep change requires the ability to disrupt and alter existing patterns of action and involves taking risks. For deep change to occur, individuals need to be open, vulnerable, and able to surrender control (ie, take on risk).

Developmental change and transformational change are 2 other types of changes. These can also occur at the individual and organizational levels. *Developmental change* occurs when you recognize a need to improve an existing situation or level of performance. In this case, whatever needs to change does not need to be recreated or reinvented, but instead, must be refined in some way to make it better. Individuals may need specific training and/or coaching if new skills are required to make the change successful.

Transformational change, a systems approach to change or change that happens at all levels, is radical, holistic, profound, deep-seated, and irreversible. Transformational change often requires you to break through paradigms, beliefs, and behavior to convert real or perceived obstacles into hopeful and exciting opportunities and new ways of interacting. Transformational change uses and emphasizes the power of a positive, shared vision that focuses on what could be possible to inspire action. Recall from Chapter 3, transformational leadership happens when both leaders and followers interact in ways that move each other to higher levels of conviction, engagement, and motivation.[7] In these dynamic leader-follower relationships, both the leader and the followers find meaning and purpose in their work, and both grow and develop from their relationship. Therefore, leading transformational change successfully relies on highly skilled, interdependent collaboration; requires a high level of commitment; and needs the collective energy to be fueled through dynamic relationships connected by a mutual purpose.

Recall also from Chapter 3, "uplifting, passionate, and energizing" describes the style of the transformational leader. These leaders demonstrate care for others; display a duty to help others succeed; and earn trust, respect, and admiration from their followers in such a way that their followers consciously choose to follow them as the leader—and that choice makes for a significant, dynamic bond.[7] Transformational leaders are proficient at leveraging the strength of their vision and personality to inspire followers to change expectations, perceptions, and motivations to work toward common goals. Transformational leaders exude energy and passion in such a way that their followers become engaged and re-engaged to keep an ongoing, high level of commitment to the vision. Their unwavering and energetic commitment motivates others, particularly through tough and challenging times.

TABLE 9-1. PLANNING FOR CHANGE	
STEP 1: LIST THE 10 MOST SIGNIFICANT PERSONAL CHANGES YOU HAVE EVER MADE.	STEP 2: CATEGORIZE EACH CHANGE AS PLANNED OR UNPLANNED, INCREMENTAL OR DEEP, AND DEVELOPMENTAL AND/OR TRANSFORMATIONAL.
1.	
2.	
3.	
4.	
5.	
6.	
7.	
8.	
9.	
10.	
STEP 3: SUMMARIZE YOUR EXPERIENCE WITH MAKING DEEP CHANGE AT THE PERSONAL LEVEL. WHAT HAS BEEN EASY ABOUT MAKING DEEP CHANGE? WHAT HAS BEEN HARD? WHY? WHAT HAS HELPED?	
STEP 4: WRITE YOUR OWN DEFINITION OF *DEEP CHANGE*.	

Personal Change

Personal change is self-change or change as an individual person. As the environment changes around you (which will happen all the time), it is possible for you to lose your sense of alignment. You may feel pushed out of your comfort zone—who you are, and how you interact with others—by forces outside your control. Often, you can make a small adjustment or an incremental change to regain your balance or sense of stability. However, you sometimes will need to alter your fundamental assumptions or paradigms and develop new ideas about yourself and your surrounding environments to do so. Making deep personal change is not easy, and it takes courage. Recall that deep change tends to be meaningful, significant in scope, multifaceted, and usually irreversible. Deep personal change requires new ways of thinking and behaving and involves taking risks. For deep personal change to occur, individuals need to be open, vulnerable, and able to surrender control (ie, take on risk).

Activity 9-3: You and Personal Change

Failing to plan for change may lead to unplanned change. Complete the items in Table 9-1 to help you start planning for change.

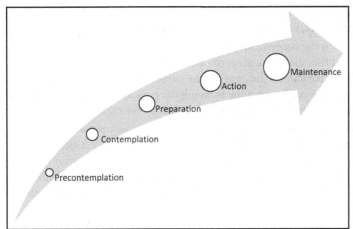

Figure 9-1. Transtheoretical Model of Change: stages of behavioral change. (Adapted from Prochaska JO, DiClemente CC, Norcross JC. In search of how people change: applications to addictive behaviors. *Am Psychol.* 1992;47[9]:1102 and Prochaska J, DiClemente C. Stages and processes of self-change in smoking: toward an integrative model of change. *J Consult Clin Psychol.* 1983;5:390-395.)

Bottom Line!

"Everyone thinks of changing the world, but no one thinks of changing himself."
– Leo Tolstoy, world-renowned Russian writer

CHANGE IS A PROCESS

Experts, studying the phenomenon of change, have proposed models of change to help individuals and organizations design, lead, manage, and facilitate effective change in different situations. These models explain change as sequences of individual and collective events, actions, and activities unfolding over time within a context.[8] Steps within the change process may include getting facts or the reasons for why the change is happening, paying attention to feelings, making explicit commitments, and taking action. Understanding the processes of change will help you become more effective in leading change and attaining desired behavioral change. The Transtheoretical Model of Change is particularly useful in helping you understand the process and decisions behind making personal behavioral change.

Transtheoretical Model of Change: Building Readiness for Change

The *Transtheoretical Model of Change* is an integrative, biopsychosocial model to conceptualize the process of intentional behavior change.[9,10] This model recognizes change as a process that unfolds over time, and suggests that (health) behavior change involves progress through distinct stages, including precontemplation, contemplation, preparation, action, and maintenance (Figure 9-1).[9,10]

Individuals often progress through these stages of change in a linear way; however, a nonlinear progression is also common. Moreover, it is not uncommon for individuals to recycle through the stages or to regress to earlier stages depending on their situations. Keep this in mind as you read through each stage in more detail.

- Precontemplation stage: You are in the precontemplation stage when you are not ready to act in the immediate future (ie, within the next 6 months). When you are in this stage, the relative cons for change overshadow the pros in favor of behavior change, and these cons help maintain existing behavior. You might also be in this stage because you do not understand the consequences your behavior is causing. Or, you might not be ready to make a change. Perhaps you do not intend to act because you have attempted to change your behavior unsuccessfully, and these failed attempts have left you discouraged about your ability to change.

- Contemplation stage: If you are in the contemplation stage, you are getting ready to change (ie, within in the next 6 months). At this stage, you are more aware of the pros or benefits of changing your behavior, but you are also aware of the cons. In the contemplation stage, the pros and cons tend to carry equal weight. You might continue to weigh the pros against the cons, yet this analysis paralysis can cause you to procrastinate or be ambivalent toward taking action.

- Preparation stage: When the pros in favor of changing outweigh the cons for maintaining certain behavior, you move to the preparation or sometimes directly to the action stage. If you are in the preparation stage, then you are ready to act in the immediate future (ie, within the next month). Typically, you have already taken some important action in the past several months. For example, you have established your plan of action, such as joining a gym, buying workout clothes, or finding healthful menus to try.

- Action stage: If you are in the action stage, then you have made specific overt and meaningful modifications in your lifestyle within the past 6 months.

- Maintenance stage: As you enter the maintenance stage, the pros in favor of maintaining the behavior change should outweigh any cons of reverting to old behaviors. If you are in the maintenance stage, then you have made specific overt and meaningful modifications in your lifestyle and are working to prevent relapse. While in this stage, you are less tempted to relapse into old patterns of behavior, and you grow increasingly more confident in your ability to sustain your lifestyle changes.

A-HA! – ARE YOU READY TO MAKE A CHANGE?

Write down a personal behavior change you have wanted to make for some time but have not made yet. Examples may include losing 10 pounds, exercising more, journaling more, eating less or eating better, drinking less, or quitting smoking.

_____

_____

_____

Why you have not changed your behavior yet?

_____

_____

_____

Using the Transtheoretical Model of Change steps described previously, which stage of change are you in based on what you stated above?

_____

_____

_____

●————————————

Transitioning Through Change

Change happens to you, even if you do not want it to happen or agree with it. Transition, on the other hand, is internal; it is what happens in your mind and heart as you progress through change.

Transition is the inner psychological process that people go through as they internalize and come to terms with the new situation that the change brings about.[11] The starting point for dealing with transition is the endings that people have to face to let go and move forward. Change can happen quickly, while transition usually occurs slowly. One model developed by Bridges highlights 3 stages of transition that people experiencing change go through, including Endings (stage 1), Neutral Zone (stage 2), and New Beginnings (stage 3).[11] Bridges claims that people go through each stage at their own pace. For example, if you are comfortable with change, then you may move ahead to stage 3 quickly, while others may linger at stages 1 or 2.

1. Stage 1: Endings
   ◦ You enter this first stage of transition when change presents itself. You may experience resistance and emotional turmoil because you are being compelled to let go of something you might be comfortable with or used to doing. Furthermore, at this stage, you may experience a range of emotions including fear, denial, anger, sadness, disorientation, frustration, uncertainty, and a sense of loss. As part of this transition, you have to accept that something is ending before you can begin to accept any new opportunity or challenge.

2. Stage 2: The Neutral Zone
   ◦ In this stage, you may still feel attached to the old way while you are also trying to adapt to the new way. You may feel confused, uncertain, and impatient. You may even experience resentment toward the change initiative; low morale and low productivity; anxiety about your role, status, or identity; and skepticism about the change initiative. Depending on how well the change is progressing, you may also experience a higher workload as you get used to new systems and new ways of working.

3. Stage 3: New Beginnings
   ◦ The last transition stage is a time of acceptance and energy. You begin to embrace the change initiative. You are building the skills you need to work successfully in the new way, and you are starting to see early wins from your efforts. At this stage, you are likely to experience high energy, openness to learning, and renewed commitment to the group or your role.

A-HA! – DO YOU GET STUCK?

Change happens to you, even if you do not want it or agree with it. Transition is internal; it is what happens in your mind and heart as you progress through change.

What was the last big change that occurred in your life?

_____

How was your transition to the new beginning following that change? As a self-reflection process, review steps 1 to 3 above, and describe how long you felt you spent in each of the stages.

_____
_____
_____

Would you describe this as a typical transition process for you, or have other circumstances or changes had different responses in you?

_____
_____
_____

Resistance to Change

Change can be uncomfortable for many reasons, and this discomfort can fuel resistance, sometimes unintentionally. *Resistance to change* is the act of opposing or struggling with anything that alters the status quo. Resistance can be covert or overt, and organized or individual. Individuals may discover that they do not like or want to change and may resist publicly, verbally, or aggressively. Resistance to change may appear in actions such as verbal criticism, nitpicking details, loud and verbal failure to adapt, snide comments, sarcastic remarks, missed meetings, failed commitments, endless arguments, lack of support verbally, and even outright sabotage. Covert resistance to change is usually not visible, demonstrated, or expressed openly.

There are many reasons why resistance to change exists. For example, resistance may develop when misunderstandings arise about the need for change, the reasons for change are not clear, or people believe strongly that the current way of doing things works well. One of the most common reasons for resistance is fear of the unknown. People will only take active steps toward the unknown if they genuinely believe or feel the risks of maintaining the status quo are greater than the risks of moving forward. People may fear they lack the skills or ability to perform effectively in a new way. Letting go of old habits, routines, and past memories may cause resistance to change.

In leading change, it is important to accept that resistance to change exists, and that change processes trigger emotional reactions. Allowing time for people let go, accept change, and express their feelings can help facilitate change or movement in the right direction. People often fear what they do not understand; therefore, the more you can educate yourself and others about a positive future, and communicate how their knowledge and skills are an essential part of getting there, the higher the probability they will move to the next stage. When people are engaged—as early as possible—as part of the change process, then there is less resistance.

A-HA! – BREAKING THROUGH THE BARRIER OF RESISTANCE

The Transtheoretical Model of Change is used to build readiness for change by overcoming resistance. *Change readiness* means all the obstacles that prevent you from changing have been removed, so the only thing left for you to do is change! Review your responses in the A-Ha! – Are You Ready to Make a Change? segment on page 170.

Identify 3 specific actions you could take to facilitate the change you want to make (to stop yourself from resisting change).

_____

_____

_____

●————————————

LEADING CHANGE

What does it take to lead change and make change happen? A *change agent* is a person who acts as a catalyst to help an organization transform itself by initiating and championing the change process. To be effective, the change agent focuses on the people in the organization and their interactions. Kotter recommends the following 8 steps for change agents to follow in implementing fundamental organizational change[12]:

1. Establishing a sense of urgency
2. Forming a coalition of individuals who embrace the need for change and who can rally others to support the effort

3. Creating a vision to accomplish the desired result
4. Communicating the vision through numerous communication channels
5. Empowering others to act on the vision to facilitate implementation
6. Creating short-term wins by publicizing success, thereby building momentum for continued change
7. Consolidating improvements and changing other structures, systems, procedures, and policies not consistent with the vision
8. Institutionalizing the new approaches by publicizing the connection between the change effort and organizational success

Kotter's first 5 phases align somewhat with Lewin's unfreezing stage (planned change), providing another perspective about the importance of preparing for change. Moreover, understanding an organization's culture, as revealed in its rules, policies, customs, norms, ceremonies, and rewards, is important in a change process.[13]

The information and activities in this book so far have led you toward being an effective change agent. Having a clear vision, patience and persistence, assertiveness and an ability to ask tough questions, knowledge and access to information, an ability to lead by example, and a network of strong relationships built on trust have all been highlighted. Ironically, change agents need those exact characteristics to be effective catalysts of change.

A-HA! – YOU CAN BE A CHANGE AGENT

Identify one change you would like to help facilitate at the clinical or organizational level.

_____

Why is this change important to you?

_____

Review the list of change agent characteristics. Identify the key characteristics that you will need for this particular change that you want to make.

_____

What skills, if any, do you feel you need to develop further before initiating this change?

_____

_____

Bottom Line!

"You must be the change you want to see in the world." – Mahatma Gandhi, Indian civil rights activist

Even though life changes are predictable, you can initiate personal change proactively to develop your personal leadership skills and become a better person as a result. There is always potential to lead positive change in every interaction, in every situation, and at all levels of clinical practice.

Case Study: Diane E. Clark's Story

Reread the Leadership Vignette presented at the beginning of this chapter. This case study represents the story of physical therapist Diane E. Clark, who led change as a change agent within a doctor of physical therapy program. According to Clark's story:

- Why is it important for us to lead change in physical therapy?
- Why is leading change difficult?
- What makes leading change easier?
- What makes leading change difficult?
- What role does the change agent or change champion play in leading change?

CHAPTER KEY WORDS

Change, Planned Change, Unplanned Change, Incremental Change, Deep Change, Developmental Change, Transformational Change, Personal Change, Transition, Change Readiness, Change Agent, Resistance to Change

REFERENCES

1. Kouzes JM, Posner BZ. *The Leadership Challenge: How to Make Extraordinary Things Happen in Organizations.* 6th ed. Somerset, NJ: John Wiley & Sons, Incorporated; 2017.

2. Sinek S. *Start with Why: How Great Leaders Inspire Everyone to Take Action.* London, UK: Penguin; 2009.

3. Mindtools. *How Confident Are You? Self-Assessment.* https://www.mindtools.com/pages/article/newTCS_84.htm. Accessed August 23, 2018.

4. American Psychological Association. *The road to resilience.* https://www.apa.org/topics/resilience. Accessed September 25, 2018.

5. Watson G. Resistance to change. *Am Behav Sci.* 1971;14(5):745-766.

6. Lewin K. Frontiers in group dynamics. In: *Field Theory in Social Science.* London, UK: Social Science Paperbacks; 1947.

7. Burns JM, Frank and Virginia Williams Collection of Lincolniana (Mississippi State University. Libraries). Leadership. New York, NY: Harper & Row; 1979.

8. Ford MW, Greer BM. Profiling change: an empirical study of change process patterns. *J Appl Behav Sci.* 2006;42(4):420-446. doi:10.1177/0021886306293437

9. Prochaska JO, DiClemente CC, Norcross JC. In search of how people change: applications to addictive behaviors. *Am Psychol.* 1992;47(9):1102.

10. Prochaska J, DiClemente C. Stages and processes of self-change in smoking: toward an integrative model of change. *J Consult Clin Psychol.* 1983;5:390-395.

11. Bridges W. *Transitions: Making Sense of Life's Changes.* Cambridge, MA: Da Capo Press; 2004.

12. Kotter JP. *Leading Change.* Brighton, MA: Harvard Business Press; 2012.

13. Galpin TJ. *The Human Side of Change: A Practical Guide to Organization Redesign.* Hoboken, NJ: Wiley; 1996.

SUGGESTED READINGS

Heath C, Heath D. *Switch: How to Change Things When Change is Hard.* New York, NY: Broadway Books; 2010.

Kotter JP. *Leading Change.* Boston, MA: Harvard Business School Press; 1996.

10

Ethical Leadership and Decision Making

Nancy R. Kirsch, PT, DPT, PhD, FAPTA

Ethics is not about the way things are, it is about the way things ought to be.
— Michael Josephson, law professor, attorney, and founder of the Josephson Institute of Ethics

CHAPTER OBJECTIVES

› Apply the 6 ethical principles to cases discussed in class.
› Identify the appropriate principle or standard to provide guidance in a case analysis.
› Appreciate the need for a higher moral standard for health care providers over the general public.
› Apply the Realm-Individual Process-Situation ethical analysis model to clinical cases.
› Recognize the need for moral courage and moral potency in carrying out an ethical action.

Green-Wilson J, Zeigler S, eds.
Learning to Lead in Physical Therapy (pp 175-192).
© 2020 Taylor & Francis Group.

Leadership Vignette

Laura Lee (Dolly) Swisher, PT, MDiv, PhD, FNAP, FAPTA

I cannot point to any one person or event that stimulated my interest in ethical decision making. I believe my interest in ethical decision making is partly based on who I am, but was also reinforced by my parents and family. My parents often discussed ethical issues, and looking back, I would say my father lived out his ethical convictions and was a good model of virtue. However, several people, social occurrences, and personal factors influenced my interest in the subject of ethics. As a baby boomer, I think of the effects of World War II (WWII). My father served in the Army Air Corps. Like others, he enlisted to protect the United States, but his generation perceived WWII as a moral war. The aftermath posed many ethical questions. As our knowledge of the fate of Jewish people, gay people, and gypsies in the Nazi camps spread, children in my generation were confronted with and discussed how good people could face profound evil. Note that even members of the medical profession participated in these atrocities.

The events of WWII stimulated the work of both Kohlberg and Milgram. Although Kohlberg examined how moral thinking developed, Milgram was interested in how people respond to authority in promoting or stopping harm (Box 10-1).[1]

To some extent, I believe that Milgram's experiment (ironically an experiment that might be considered unethical by today's standards) demonstrated that each of us must be a leader on ethical matters or when confronted with danger. I was profoundly influenced by the leadership of Martin Luther King Jr and the courage of the freedom riders that engaged in nonviolent protests of social injustices. Their actions were powerful indicators that recognizing the right thing to do was not enough: one must also act. Unfortunately, ethics is often taught and analyzed in isolation from clinical, managerial, leadership, or even personal issues. Yet, in reality, ethics is a dimension of everything we do. Every professional must lead ethically; no aspect of anyone's professional life is completely void of moral import. To lead is to influence others through trustworthy relationships, power, positional or formal authority, words, or example, and from this perspective, each of us has some opportunity to be a leader. One of the core issues that professionals face is what to do when an authoritative leader asks them to engage in unethical behavior. Every professional, regardless of whether he or she is a front-line therapist or the chief operating officer, is called to lead by speaking up and stepping forth. The quandary of moral silence is portrayed eloquently in this statement from a poem written by Martin Niemoller, prominent German anti-Nazi theologian and Lutheran pastor, best known as the author of the poem *First they came...*[2]:

> *First they came for the socialists, and I did not speak out—*
> *Because I was not a socialist.*
> *Then they came for the trade unionists, and I did not speak out—*
> *Because I was not a trade unionist.*
> *Then they came for the Jews, and I did not speak out—*
> *Because I was not a Jew.*
> *Then they came for me—and there was no one left to speak for me.*

It is important to develop a personal and systematic process to carefully examine difficult ethical issues. What do you do when faced with a difficult choice or situation, or moral ambiguity or uncertainty? The literature suggests that physical therapists may not use a systematic process, look at the ethics literature, or consult colleagues in resolving ethical dilemmas. This is interesting because most physical therapists would approach clinical issues using a systematic process, based on existing evidence, and in consultation with wiser colleagues. A sound process and possible ethics mentors could be helpful resources.

Focus on success is easy; it is tempting to believe that one will do the right thing. However, the truth is that at some time in our lives, each of us will fail to fulfill our own high ethical ideals in the personal or professional arena. Learn from moral failures. Analyzing failure requires personal moral courage, and moral courage is fundamental to leadership.

Box 10-1

THE MILGRAM EXPERIMENT

Stanley Milgram conducted the Milgram experiment on obedience to authority figures. These experiments (which began in July 1961, 3 months after the start of the trial of German Nazi war criminal Adolf Eichmann) measured the willingness of study participants to obey a figure of authority who instructed them to perform acts that conflicted with their personal conscience.

The experimenter ordered the teacher, who was the subject of the experiment, to give what the teacher believed were painful electric shocks to a learner, who was an actor. The subject/teacher believed that the learner was receiving actual electric shocks for each wrong answer, though in reality there were no such punishments. Being separated from the subject/teacher, the learner/actor set up a tape recorder integrated with the electroshock generator, which played prerecorded sounds for each shock level. After a number of voltage level increases, the actor started to bang on the wall that separated him from the subject/teacher. After banging several times on the wall and complaining about a heart condition, the learner would cease all responses. At this point, many people indicated their desire to stop the experiment and check on the learner. Some test subjects paused at 135 volts and began to question the purpose of the experiment. Most continued after being assured that they would not be held responsible. A few subjects began to laugh nervously or exhibit other signs of extreme stress once they heard the screams of pain coming from the learner.

The extreme willingness of adults to go to almost any lengths on the command of an authority constitutes the chief finding of this study. In Milgram's first set of experiments, 65% (26 of 40) of experiment participants administered the experiment's final massive 450-volt shock, though many were uncomfortable doing so; at some point, every participant paused and questioned the experiment, and some said they would refund the money they were paid for participating in the experiment. Throughout the experiment, subjects displayed varying degrees of tension and stress. Subjects were sweating, trembling, stuttering, biting their lips, groaning, or digging their fingernails into their skin, and some were even having nervous laughing fits or seizures.

Reprinted with permission from Milgram S. Behavioral study of obedience. *J Abnorm Soc Psychol.* 1963;67(4):371.

ETHICAL LEADERSHIP AND YOU

Ethics can be described as a systematic analysis of morals and behavior, or how individuals act during their personal and professional undertakings.[3] Potter Stewart, a former Associate Justice of the US Supreme Court, claims, "Ethics is knowing the difference between what you have a right to do and what is right to do."[4] A leader today must have a strong and well-defined ethical or moral compass to succeed in life, practice, and the profession. A set of stable core beliefs is essential for any leader (starting with personal leadership; refer to Chapter 1) to respond ethically to the range of complex issues that will be encountered in personal and professional life. This chapter focuses on the value of ethical leadership, how to develop ethical leadership skills, and how you can make effective ethical decisions as a personal leader in daily practice.

A-HA! – YOUR PERSONAL ETHICS

Select and reflect upon an experience in which your personal ethics were challenged. Describe how these were challenged.

_____

_____

_____

What factors did you consider when selecting this experience to reflect upon?

_____

_____

_____

How did you respond to this challenge?

_____

_____

_____

Did you use leadership skills to make positive change from this experience? Why or why not?

_____

_____

_____

To be seen as an ethical leader, you and others must perceive ethical aspects of your leadership.[5] According to Piccolo et al, ethical leaders capture employees' perceptions of the ethical behavior inferred from the leader's conduct.[6] Developing a reputation for ethical leadership rests upon the 2 pillars of moral being and moral managing.[5] _Moral being_ relates to being an ethical person, and one who consistently makes decisions and acts based on a foundational set of ethical values. _Moral managing_ pertains to the process of creating perceptions in others, such as the importance of ethics and values in the organization, and how individuals practice on a daily basis.[5] Leaders demonstrate ethical awareness by being attentive to the collective good of the group, understanding the impact of both the process to be used, identifying the long- and short-term outcomes, and knowing the perspectives and interests of stakeholders.

TABLE 10-1. PERCEIVED LEADER INTEGRITY SCALE SELF-ASSESSMENT (ADAPTED)

Directions: Circle responses to indicate how well each item describes the person you are assessing, using the following response choices:

SAMPLE STATEMENTS/QUESTIONS	NOT AT ALL	SOMEWHAT	VERY MUCH	EXACTLY
Would use my mistakes to attack me personally	1	2	3	4
Always gets even	1	2	3	4
Gives special favors to certain or specific people but not to me	1	2	3	4
Would lie to me	1	2	3	4
Deliberately fuels conflict among other people	1	2	3	4
Would allow me to be blamed for his or her mistake	1	2	3	4
Makes fun of my mistakes instead of coaching me to do my job better	1	2	3	4
Would deliberately exaggerate my mistakes to make me look bad when describing my performance to others	1	2	3	4
Is vindictive	1	2	3	4
Deliberately makes others angry at each other	1	2	3	4
Would make trouble for me if I got on his or her bad side	1	2	3	4
Would take credit for my ideas	1	2	3	4
Total Score:				

Reprinted with permission from Johnson CE. *Meeting the Ethical Challenges of Leadership.* 3rd ed. Thousand Oaks, CA: Sage Publications, Inc; 2009.

Activity 10-1: Perceptions of Your Ethics and Leadership

Use the sample questions listed in Table 10-1,[7] provided from the Perceived Leader Integrity Scale Self-Assessment (adapted version), to gain feedback from your peers by asking them to rate their perceptions of you as a leader. Interpretation: The higher the score, the lower the integrity of the person rated.

Health care professionals are held to a higher standard of ethics because of the type of service they provide. They must simultaneously focus on the loyalty toward their patients and their responsibility to the priorities of the organization, while navigating the ongoing financial pressures associated with providing services in today's health care environment.[3] It is crucial for physical therapists, as health care professionals, to consider the ethical and societal responsibilities inherent in the label of being a professional, and to focus sincerely on doing what is good and right for their patients while balancing legal requirements and meeting federal regulations.[8] Often, ethics are collected and systematically organized or codified into a code of ethics or statement of behaviors expected by professional associations and to which individual professionals aspire. Physical therapy as a profession demonstrates autonomy or self-governance; inherently, this requires the profession of physical therapy to establish and enforce its code of ethics. In the physical therapy profession, there is only one accepted and articulated Code of Ethics for physical therapists, the American Physical Therapy Assocation's (APTA) *Code of Ethics for the Physical Therapist* (Code), and only one accepted and articulated set of standards for physical therapist assistants, the APTA's *Standards of Ethical Conduct for the Physical Therapist Assistant* (Standards). The APTA's 2009 House of Delegates expanded and revised these 2 core documents of the physical therapy profession, and these revisions were adopted to better delineate the ethical obligations of all physical therapists and physical therapist assistants. The APTA House of Delegates makes occasional revisions to the Code of Ethics such as the small revision in 2019.

Activity 10-2: Review the Profession's Code of Ethics

Review the APTA's *Code of Ethics for the Physical Therapist*[9] and APTA's *Standards of Ethical Conduct for the Physical Therapist Assistant*,[10] both found at http://www.apta.org/Ethics/Core.

Further your knowledge of these core documents by reviewing APTA's *Guide for Professional Conduct*[11] and *Guide for Conduct of the Physical Therapist Assistant*[12], which can also be found at http://www.apta.org/Ethics/Core.

Dickson, Resick, and Hanges identified 6 characteristics of ethical leadership, including[13]:

1. Character and integrity
2. Ethical awareness
3. Community- and people-oriented
4. Collective motivation
5. Encouraging/empowering
6. Managing ethical accountability

Do you see evidence of these 6 characteristics within the APTA *Code of Ethics*?

Do you also see your personal ethics within both of these frameworks?

It is important to emphasize that, as a health care professional, you not only have to maintain a stronger code of ethics, but you also must not cross the boundaries expected of your ethical behavior. Once society agrees to a specific code of behavior to be accepted or included in that society, all ethical decisions then require people to determine whether they will follow this code or these ethical guidelines. Specifically, you decide to behave within this code, or not. If not, then you are said to have crossed an ethical boundary. Indeed, all decisions of ethical behavior involve a question of whether you or another individual will make a choice that crosses an ethical boundary. Some ethical boundaries involve making decisions that are clearly right or wrong. These decisions usually require choosing between ethical or unethical behavior. Unfortunately, there are times when an individual is more vulnerable to making a poor ethical decision and subsequently crossing ethical boundaries. Vulnerabilities, real or perceived, can include factors such as emotional stress, mood changes, or financial instability. It is the responsibility of practicing therapists to always be self-aware and recognize when they are most vulnerable to challenges to safe and effective care.

Increased knowledge of ethical issues, decisions, and vulnerabilities can reduce unethical behaviors and boundary violations. An individual who can identify ethical conflicts, refine the ability to analyze ethical decision making appropriately, and reduce potential exposure to boundary violations, can withstand the obstacles of today's challenging ethics.

> ## Bottom Line!
>
> When health care professionals truly assume the responsibilities of leadership, they assume the unique set of ethical duties involving issues related to power, information, accountability, integrity, and responsibility. How professionals handle the innate challenges and expectations of leadership, including ethical decision making and leveraging power to influence others, determines whether they cause more harm than good.

ETHICAL PRINCIPLES

Ethical principles help physical therapists determine their *moral threshold*—the bar below which the therapist is not willing to concede without compromising integrity as a practitioner. Biomedical ethics span all practice settings, and bioethicists commonly accept 4 basic principles: autonomy, beneficence, nonmaleficence, and justice. In addition, physical therapists often speak of veracity and fidelity as foundational ethical principles, and these are added here because they are relevant to leadership and ethical decision making.

Autonomy

For many years, common medical practice essentially allowed physicians and other health care providers to make decisions for their patients. Gradually, this paternalistic approach has been replaced with patient autonomy, whereby patients and doctors share the decision-making responsibility. Consequently, doctor-patient relationships are changing. Yet, conflicts still exist as the medical community and those it serves continue to struggle to define their respective and everchanging roles.

Autonomy, in the context of medicine, allows for respect for patients' rights. Consent, particularly informed consent, is the cornerstone of patients' rights. Patients have the right to be informed of their condition, to know the risk and benefits of treatment, and to make an independent choice about their care. Specifically, the Patient Autonomy Principle 2C in the APTA's *Code of Ethics for the Physical Therapist*[9] states: "Physical therapists shall provide the information necessary to allow patients or their surrogates to make informed decisions about physical therapy care or participation in clinical research."[9]

The purpose underlying Principle 2C is to require a physical therapist to respect patient autonomy. To do so, a physical therapist must communicate to the patient/client the findings of the examination, evaluation, diagnosis, and prognosis; use sound professional judgment in informing the patient/client of any substantial risks of the recommended examination and intervention; and collaborate with the patient/client to establish the goals of treatment and the plan of care. Ultimately, a physical therapist must respect the patient's/client's right to make decisions regarding the recommended plan of care, including consent, modification, or refusal.[11]

Beneficence

The physical therapist who is a beneficent practitioner provides care that is in the best interest of the patient. However, it is not uncommon for a therapist to be caught between the demands of beneficence toward the patient and the power of patient autonomy. For example, the physical therapist determines that the most beneficial plan of care for a patient includes 3 visits per week for 2 weeks, then decreasing to twice per week. The patient declines this plan because of the very high copay, choosing to only come once per week. The therapist approaches the director about treating this patient one day per week pro bono after hours, promoting ethical leadership principles.

Nonmaleficence

Nonmaleficence means "do no harm." According to this principle, the practitioner must ask if the actions will harm the patient, either by omission or commission. "Do no harm" is strongly associated with "intend no harm." Although the physical therapist may have the best of intentions, outside influences often stand in the way between those good intentions and the institution's conflicting priorities (as will be seen in the case studies presented in this chapter). If an attempt to do no harm conflicts with the rights of the patient and autonomous decision making, vicarious harm can be done.

Justice

Justice refers to equity and fairness. The principle of justice reinforces the importance of not treating people differently based on age, gender, race, ethnicity, religion, or social status. Justice helps discern the morally best resolution to situations involving conflicts of interests, or when questions of justice or injustice arise in situations involving ethical dilemmas. Issues of justice often play out in the institutional and societal realms.[14] For example, when referring to workplace climate or atmosphere, justice means fair and impartial treatment of employees, and unbiased praise and consequences. Justice can be divided into noncomparative justice and comparative justice. *Noncomparative justice* is concerned with ensuring people get their entitlements, while comparative justice is concerned with the fair distribution of benefits and burdens in society. A form of comparative justice is *distributive justice*, which is concerned with the fair allocation of resources among diverse members of a community or society. Fair allocation typically considers the total amount of goods to be distributed, the distributing procedure, and the resulting pattern of distribution. Access to health care, or a person's ability to receive health care services when needed, is an example of distributive justice.

A-HA! – JUSTICE IN CARE

Consider this scenario: Two emergency room patients are equally in need of care, they came in at the exact same time, and both are equal in all other relevant aspects. Who should get treated first, and why? Many people feel that all people should have equal access to a basic minimal level of health care, and that a higher-level of care is the responsibility of the individual.

What do you define as a basic minimal level of care?

_____

_____

_____

Are there situations in which unequal treatment is justified, and if so, why?

_____

_____

_____

Veracity

Veracity, the principle of truthfulness, is grounded in respect for others as well as in the principle of autonomy. A person needs to have relevant information to make a decision, and this information must be clear, truthful, and understandable. However, telling the truth can be violated by lying, deliberately exchanging incorrect information, or intentionally omitting or withholding all or portions of the truth. Additionally, veracity can fail when information is disguised in jargon, in language that is intentionally misleading, or in language that does not convey the information in a way that the recipient can understand.

The following situations highlight how veracity applies to health care:

- Patients and families rely upon health care professionals for information to make informed choices about their care.
- Patients expect to be told the truth about their care, including errors or potential risks.
- Health care professionals are expected to interact with colleagues and other stakeholders with honesty while documenting, billing, conducting peer reviews, managing risk, and complying to standards and regulations.

Fidelity

Fidelity expects people to keep their promises, do what is expected of them, perform their duties, and be trustworthy. The fidelity role also expects loyalty, but associated with a specific professional designation, such as the designation of a licensed health care provider. In health care, patients expect the following actions of fidelity[15]:

- Treat them with basic respect.
- Be competent and capable of performing the duties required of your professional role.
- Adhere to a professional code of ethics.
- Follow the policies and procedures of your organization and applicable laws.
- Honor agreements made with the patient.

Ideally, both the patient and physical therapist should be loyal to each other, but the greater burden is on the therapist.[16]

Bottom Line!

Any ethical principle can become a source of an ethical dilemma. For example, at times, a commitment to the patient may not result in the best outcome for the patient. Many times, health care professionals find themselves torn among their beliefs, the patient's wants, the expectations of other health care team members, what the organizational policy dictates, and/or what the profession or the law requires.

BARRIERS TO ETHICAL LEADERSHIP

Each of the ethical principles of autonomy, beneficence, nonmaleficence, justice, veracity, and fidelity provides the physical therapist with the foundation for ethical decision making. The challenge is that many physical therapists have not developed ethical decision-making skills as keenly as their clinical decision-making skills. Historically, working under a physician's direction, physical therapists have had little exposure to the responsibility of independent ethical decision making. The expectation that physical therapists have more autonomy and more responsibility in decision making, and the realization that barriers exist to ethical leadership, increases the complexity of many decisions.

Physical therapists and other health care professionals face barriers to making ethical decisions. One common barrier is hierarchy within an organization. Physical therapists who work within certain practices and health care organizations may not be the primary decision makers, and misuse of power by formal leadership is prevalent in many modern organizations.[7] Lack of authority may contribute to a sense of powerlessness and moral distress. Another barrier for many physical therapists is that many are uncomfortable with either conflict or ambiguity. As such, some physical therapists may avoid important ethical issues altogether. Developing the skills of ethical leadership takes insight and analysis for good decision making. This applies to overcoming the barriers that physical therapists face every day.

Activity 10-3: Overcoming Barriers to Ethical Leadership

Using the information provided in Table 10-2,[7] identify ways to overcome sample barriers to ethical leadership. For each sample barrier, indicate at least one action that you as a personal leader can take to overcome the barrier and identify the ethical leadership behavior(s) that your strategy will address. In the last box, identify specific barriers to ethical leadership in your life.

Bottom Line!

Challenges to your ethics and barriers to your ability to demonstrate ethical leadership as a personal leader are inevitable. Your ability to analyze and overcome these barriers is a skill to be learned, practiced, and reflected upon.

ETHICAL DECISION MAKING

Individuals begin developing ethical decision-making skills during childhood, guided by family, teachers, coaches, religious leaders, mentors, friends, and, ultimately, colleagues. In each of these communities, the tools are somewhat different and not necessarily transparent to the user. As students transition to a professional work environment, the demands of ethical decision making are higher, consistent with the privilege of being a health care provider. The public expects health care providers to make ethical decisions guided by a well-prescribed set of professional standards.[17,18] As practitioners transition to supervisors, they are expected to become more proficient in their ethical decision-making skills; the highest expectations are placed on the leaders who are assuming formal roles as these positions are exposed to the most opportunities to demonstrate ethical decision-making skills.

Many ethical decision-making tools are available, and most have certain structural elements in common. Park reviewed 20 ethical decision-making tools and developed an integrated model consisting of 6 steps[19]:

1. Identify an ethical problem.
2. Collect additional information to identify the problem and develop solutions.
3. Develop alternatives for analysis and comparison.
4. Select the best alternatives and justification.
5. Develop diverse, practical ways to implement ethical decisions and actions.
6. Evaluate the effects and development of strategies to prevent a similar occurrence.

The subjects in Park's study confirmed the findings of others that having a tool to use as a framework for decision making increases the confidence of the user.[17,20,21] Every tool has restrictions in its applicability, and the guidance provided by the profession's core documents, although valuable and applicable, also have limitations. Because every situation is unique, the ethical decision-making model and the core documents are applied with an appreciation of the uniqueness of each situation. These situations are generally ones in which there may be great sensitivity that all parties must be aware of during the entire process.

For example, in your facility, you have a late arrival policy that states if patients are 10 minutes late for an appointment, they will not be treated; this policy was put in place so patients would not infringe on the rights of other patients. This policy is consistent with Principle 2 that states a physical

TABLE 10-2. OVERCOMING BARRIERS TO ETHICAL LEADERSHIP

BARRIER TO ETHICAL LEADERSHIP	PERSONAL LEADERSHIP ACTION ITEM(S)	ETHICAL LEADERSHIP BEHAVIOR					
		Autonomy	*Justice*	*Beneficence*	*Nonmaleficence*	*Veracity*	*Fidelity*
You face an established culture of unethical leadership upon assuming new employment.	*Example:* 1. Analyze the culture of unethical behavior.		X				
	2. Collaborate with peers or team members and staff to design guidelines for an ethical community.	X	X	X			
	3. Facilitate peer/team member acceptance of guidelines for an ethical community and hold one another accountable.						X
A peer inaccurately records her work schedule and productivity at the end of the day.	1. 2. 3.						
Senior administration has reduced the budget, and, in your opinion, quality of service cannot be maintained.	1. 2. 3.						
Although the service was provided in a group, you are instructed to bill for individual, one-on-one care to increase revenue.	1. 2. 3.						
Identify YOUR barriers to becoming an ethical leader: • Internal? (within you) • External? (environmental) • Related to specific site or context • Conceptual or philosophical							

therapist will be trustworthy and compassionate in addressing the rights and needs of patients and clients. You have no difficulty enforcing this policy, except for your patients who are transported from a group home who have to rely on a transportation service that is frequently late. If the policy is applied to them and they are never seen, will Principle 2 be upheld and respected for them? Is there perhaps another resolution? In this case, application of the ethical decision-making model must account for all circumstances. All models must be flexible enough to account for the variability of situations.

The Realm-Individual Process-Situation (RIPS) model developed by Swisher, Arslanian, and Davis includes the 6 steps of the integrated model for decision making.[22] It recognizes that the issues that confront physical therapists range from simple situations easily managed using professional ethical standards and values to complex scenarios with competing values that can be equally compelling. The foundation of the RIPS model is the work of Glaser, who identified 3 realms in which ethical issues can potentially occur[23]:

1. Individual realm

2. Institutional/organizational realm

3. Societal realm

These realms require equal attention in the ethical decision-making process. The individual realm deals with the least complex problems as it focuses on the good of the patient/client and on the rights, duties, relationships, and behaviors among individuals.

The second realm, the institutional/organizational realm, focuses on the good of the organization and on the structures and systems that facilitate achieving organizational or institutional goals. The institution/organization realm introduces another factor in that decision making must also consider the demands of the organization. An example of the impact on the therapist decision-making process occurs when a decision about patient care impacts the clinical decision making of the therapist. A frail patient in your facility, to recover from the debilitation that occurred following surgery, is placed in an ultra-high treatment category. The therapist quickly realizes that the patient cannot tolerate the treatment required but is not permitted to decrease the treatment time because then the facility would not be able to justify the inpatient stay in the subacute facility.

Finally, the third realm of the RIPS model, the societal realm, deals with the most complex issues because it is concerned with the common good or the well-being of an entire society. The societal realm recognizes that an issue may have implications beyond the impact on the individual and institution. The therapist is managing limited resources for patients, such as time that can be spent with an individual patient, and decides to see a patient who needs additional time during the therapist's lunch hour. This care is not billed for, nor documented. The patient does very well as a result of this additional therapy time. However, from the societal perspective, the perception is that the original allotted time was appropriate for the patient as demonstrated by the good outcomes achieved. An unrealistic expectation is now established, and the implications for future resource allocations are profound. Why, in the future, should additional time be allotted when a very good outcome was achieved? Lower time allocations become the norm based on inaccurate data, which was the result of the therapist just trying to "do good."

After the realm is determined, the RIPS model guides the clinician to look at the individual process. The work of James Rest categorized these behaviors into 4 equally important moral components that make up the individual process of the RIPS model[24]:

1. Moral sensitivity: Purtilo described this concept as the recognition that a problem exists.

2. Moral judgment: Rest went beyond recognition, defining *moral judgment* as that which helps the individual determine between right and wrong.

3. Moral motivation: Moral values must be above all other values.

4. Moral courage: This involves the ability to determine what the most appropriate action should be and, theoretically, to act on that situation.

A deficiency in any one of the 4 components of the individual process could result in moral failure, with the inability to act. Physical therapists have shown consistent growth in all areas of ethical decision making, except moral courage. This is the most difficult area in which to take action because of conflicting thoughts about disclosure, tattling, whistle-blowing, and fact-checking before having the moral courage to report a peer or another coworker. Unfortunately, many health care providers are dealing with inconsistent levels of effective and accurate reporting.

Hannah and Avolio claim that people need *moral potency*, defined as "the capacity to generate responsibility and motivation to take moral action in the face of adversity and persevere through challenges."[25(p 295)] They identify 3 components as constituting moral potency: moral ownership, moral efficacy, and moral courage.[25,26] Arising from one's level of moral ownership is the capacity to feel and show a sense of responsibility to take ethical action when faced with ethical issues. Even though someone has made a sound moral judgment and perhaps feels ownership to act, that person still may not act due to a lack of confidence in personal capabilities to organize, mobilize, and develop solutions to ethical issues or to confront a peer or superior. To act, individuals require moral courage or character strength to face threats and overcome fears.[25,26] Research has demonstrated that moral potency can be shaped and developed, and overall, it has been positively related to ethical behaviors, pro-social behaviors, and intentions to report others' unethical actions; negatively related to tolerance for the mistreatment of others; and enhanced by authentic and ethical leadership, as well as the ethical culture of one's organization.[25,27]

Activity 10-4: Your Moral Potency

Hannah and Avolio have developed a Moral Potency Questionnaire (MPQ).[28] Ratings have been shown to predict ethical attitudes and behaviors, and can be used as a reflection tool for your actions to support your growth in the area of moral compass. The MPQ is proprietary with a minimal fee. Sample questions are available for free on the MPQ website[28]: https://www.mindgarden.com/121-moral-potency-questionnaire#horizontalTab1

Take the full MPQ, or at least answer the sample questions available through the Mind Garden website.

The final component of the RIPS model to assist the leader in making an ethical decision is to identify the ethical situation. The practitioner must consider the following questions:

- Is this an ethical problem? An *ethical problem* is a challenge or threat to the individual's moral values.
- Is this ethical distress? Ethical distress focuses on the practitioners, in that they know the action they should take, but there is a barrier to doing what is right.
- Is this an ethical dilemma? An ethical dilemma is a problem that involves 2 or more morally correct courses of action, both of which cannot be followed. When one course of action is chosen over another, the practitioner may be doing something right and wrong at the same time.
- Is this an ethical temptation? Ethical temptation evolves from having 2 courses of action: one is morally correct, and the other is morally incorrect. If the incorrect action is chosen, silence occurs when the problem is ignored and no action is taken. The concept of moral potency evolves out of the situations that evolve from ethical silence.

Bottom Line!

There are many models for ethical decision making. The RIPS model presented in this chapter permits the clinician to quickly weigh the components of ethical decision making and integrate them with the clinical decision making for that patient.

Case Study: Challenging Leadership—Tim

Tim had been working at Star Physical Therapy for more than 1 year. He loved the patient population. His coworkers were supportive, and everyone worked well together. One Friday at the weekly staff meeting, George, the practice owner, and his wife, Amanda, the office manager, presented a new treatment protocol. George said that he had been doing some reading, and it appeared that the benefits of ultrasound outweighed the risks. He encouraged the staff to begin using ultrasound with every patient. Bob, one of the senior therapists, asked for some clarification: "encouraged" or "required?" George chuckled and told Bob that he certainly could make his own treatment decisions, but George expected to see the volume of ultrasound increase accordingly. Tim found the discussion interesting, but it did not apply to his patients. He quickly assessed his caseload and realized that he could not justify using ultrasound to treat a single patient. He also made a mental note that, when he asked George for specifics about the references upon which George had based his decision, his question was put off until "later." George indicated in the meeting that they would track patient outcomes for a clinical trial. Tim noticed in the following weeks that ultrasound use seemed to increase, but he was not concerned by it, and he continued to have the greatest respect for his colleagues.

Three weeks after the meeting, one of Tim's patients questioned him about the bill he had recently received from Star Physical Therapy. The bill reflected a charge for an ultrasound, but the patient had no idea what that was or when he might have received it. Tim replied that it was an error, thanked the patient for bringing it to his attention, and assured him he would handle the correction. At lunch that day, Tim approached Amanda with a copy of the bill and pointed out the error. She directed him to George for clarification. George told Tim not to worry, and that he would make sure that it was resolved, which relieved Tim. His patient notes did not mention ultrasound, and he realized that the charge for an ultrasound when it was not indicated was fraudulent. Tim assured his patient the error had been corrected. A few weeks later, Tim got a call from the same patient, who had been recently discharged. Tim expected the call to be about his patient's home program or advice on the purchase of exercise equipment. However, the call was to inform Tim that not only had his bill not been corrected, but he had also been billed for additional ultrasound charges.

Tim went directly to George, and this time requested to see his patient's billing record, which revealed at least 12 ultrasound charges. Tim confronted George and confirmed that the charges occurred both before and after their previous discussion. George reassured Tim that billing was an administrative concern, and not to worry about it. George went on to further say that Tim was not responsible for the bills, and once George had told everybody to use ultrasound on every patient, he had fully expected that all staff would comply. After all, Tim was always talking about making sure evidence was used when treating patients. George was a mentor to Tim, and Tim appreciated all that George had done for him, but he now realized that perhaps George was condoning fraudulent billing. Did George really tell Tim not to concern himself with billing? Wasn't the responsibility of the physical therapist to bill accurately clearly in the practice act? Tim needed to think about this. What was he missing? None of the other staff seemed concerned. He realized there must be an explanation that made sense, and it was just his inexperience that triggered this doubt about what was happening. Certainly, these could not all be billing errors, and of course it could not possibly be fraudulent behavior, not here!

In a discussion with a colleague about the matter, Tim felt worse. His colleague explained that maximizing reimbursement was approached in many ways. It was highly unlikely Tim would get caught, and since the boss seemed fine with it, why was Tim so concerned? This explanation revealed to Tim that his coworker was also aware of the issue, but he deliberately chose to ignore it and encouraged Tim to do so as well.

Tim had made a good effort to work within the structure of the company, but he could not justify these actions. Though he was happy at this practice setting and grateful for everything he had learned, he decided to leave and seek employment elsewhere. He could not trust the moral character of the practice leadership. He briefly considered whether the decision to leave was enough. Did he have another obligation, such as a duty to report fraudulent behavior? He was not ready to make that decision, recognizing that it would implicate his supervisor as well as his colleagues. Although he did not condone their actions, he appreciated the knowledge and guidance they had provided in his clinical development.

Tim used a multi-step method in determining the action he was going to take. Apply the RIPS Model by completing Table 10-3[22] from Tim's frame of reference.

TABLE 10-3. RIPS MODEL WORKSHEET

STEP 1: RECOGNIZE AND DEFINE THE ETHICAL ISSUE (WHICH REALMS AND SITUATIONS ARE AFFECTED)

Realm	Individual Process	Situation
Individual	Moral sensitivity	Ethical problem
Organizational	Moral judgment	Ethical distress
Societal	Moral motivation	Ethical dilemma
	Moral courage	Ethical temptation
		Silence

STEP 2: REFLECT

What are the relevant facts and contextual information?
Who are the major stakeholders?
What are the consequences (intended/unintended)?
What are the laws, duties, obligations, and ethical principles?
What professional resources may be helpful when working through an ethical problem?
How does the situation do when tested as right vs wrong?

STEP 3: DECIDE THE RIGHT THING TO DO

Rules-based	
Ends-based	
Care-based	

STEP 4: IMPLEMENT, EVALUATE, AND RE-ASSESS

Adapted from Swisher LL, Arslanian LE, Davis CM. The Realm Individual Process-Situation (RIPS) Model of ethical decision-making. *HPA Resource.* 2005;5(3).

Chapter Key Words

Ethics, Autonomy, Beneficence, Nonmaleficence, Justice, Distributive Justice, Veracity, Fidelity, Realm-Individual Process Situation (RIPS) Model, Moral Potency

References

1.   Milgram S. Behavioral study of obedience. *J Abnorm Soc Psychol.* 1963;67(4):371.

2.   Niemoller M. First they came... *US Holocaust Memorial Museum.* https://en.wikipedia.org/wiki/First_they_came_... Accessed July 28, 2019.

3.   Scott RW. *Professional Ethics: A Guide for Rehabilitation Professionals.* St. Louis, MO: Mosby; 1998.

4.   BrainyQuote.com. *Potter Stewart Quotes.* https://www.brainyquote.com/quotes/potter_stewart_390058. Accessed March 28, 2020.

5.   Trevino LK, Hartman LP, Brown M. Moral person and moral manager: how executives develop a reputation for ethical leadership. *Calif Manage Rev.* 2000;42(4):128(15).

6.   Piccolo RF, Greenbaum R, den Hartog DN, Folger R. The relationship between ethical leadership and core job characteristics. *J Organ Behav.* 2010;31(2/3):259. doi:10.1002/job.627

7.   Johnson CE. *Meeting the Ethical Challenges of Leadership.* 3rd ed. Thousand Oaks, CA: Sage Publications; 2009.

8.   Scott RW, Petrosino C, Cooperman J. *Physical Therapy Management.* St. Louis, MO: Mosby/Elsevier; 2008.

9.   American Physical Therapy Association. *Code of Ethics for the Physical Therapist.* http://www.apta.org/Ethics/Core. Accessed November 2, 2018.

10.   American Physical Therapy Association. *Standards of Ethical Conduct for the Physical Therapist Assistant.* http://www.apta.org/Ethics/Core. Accessed November 2, 2018.

11.   American Physical Therapy Association. *Guide for Professional Conduct.* http://www.apta.org/Ethics/Core. Accessed November 2, 2018.

12.   American Physical Therapy Association. *Guide for Conduct of the Physical Therapist Assistant.* http://www.apta.org/Ethics/Core. Accessed November 2, 2018.

13.   Dickson MW, Resick CJ, Hanges PJ. When organizational climate is unambiguous, it is also strong. *J Appl Psychol.* 2006;91(2):351.

14.   Gabard DL, Martin MW. *Physical Therapy Ethics.* Philadelphia, PA: FA Davis; 2003.

15.   Purtilo RB. Ethics teaching in allied health fields. *Hastings Cent Rep.* 1978;8(2):14. doi:10.2307/3560399

16.   Beauchamp TL, Childress JF. *Principles of Biomedical Ethics.* Oxford, UK: Oxford University Press; 2001.

17.   Barnett J, Behnke S, Rosenthal S, Koocher G. In case of ethical dilemma, break glass. Commentary on ethical decision making in practice. *Prof Psychol Res Pract.* 2005;38(1):7-12.

18.   Carpenter C. Moral distress in physical therapy practice. *Physiother Theory Pract.* 2010;26(2):69-78.

19.   Park EJ. An integrated ethical decision-making model for nurses. *Nurs Ethics.* 2012;19(1):139-159. doi:10.1177/0969733011413491

20.   Detert JR, Resick CJ, Hanges PJ. Moral disengagement in EDM: a study of antecedents and outcomes. *J Appl Psychol.* 2006;9(2):351-364.

21.   Eckles RE, Meslin EM, Gaffney M, Helft PR. Medical ethics education: where are we? Where should we be going? A review. *Acad Med.* 2005;80(12):1143-1152.

22.   Swisher LL, Arslanian LE, Davis CM. The Realm Individual Process-Situation (RIPS) Model of ethical decision making. *HPA Resour.* 2005;5(3).

23.   Glaser JW. *Three Realms of Ethics: Individual, Institutional, Societal.* London, UK: Sheed and Ward Publishing; 1994.

24.   Rest JR, Narveaz D. *Moral Development in the Professions: Psychology and Applied Ethics.* East Sussex, UK: Psychology Press; 1994.

25.   Hannah ST, Avolio BJ. Moral potency: building the capacity for character-based leadership. *Consult Psychol J Pract Res.* 2010;62(4):291-310.

26.   Hannah ST, Avolio BJ, May DR. Moral maturation and moral conation: a capacity approach to explaining moral thought and action. *Acad Manage Rev.* 2011;36(4):663-685.

27. Hannah ST, Avolio BJ, Walumbwa FO. Relationships between authentic leadership, moral courage, and ethical and pro-social behaviors. *Bus Ethics Q.* 2011;21(4):555-578.

28. Hannah ST, Avolio BJ. Moral Potency Questionnaire. *Mind Garden.* https://www.mindgarden.com/121-moral-potency-questionnaire#horizontalTab1. Accessed November 2, 2018.

SUGGESTED READING

Kirsch N. *Ethics in Physical Therapy: A Case Based Approach.* McGraw Hill: New York, NY; 2018.

11

Leading by Serving

Barbara A. Tschoepe, PT, DPT, PhD, FAPTA
Jennifer Green-Wilson, PT, MBA, EdD

The servant-leader is servant first… It begins with the natural feeling that one wants to serve, to serve first. Then conscious choice brings one to aspire to lead.

— *Robert K. Greenleaf, founder of the modern servant leadership movement*

CHAPTER OBJECTIVES

- ‣ Define *social responsibility*.
- ‣ Discuss how social responsibility and physical therapists are related.
- ‣ Examine a socially responsible leadership style.
- ‣ Define *social entrepreneurship* as an approach to leadership.
- ‣ Examine how advocacy, leadership, and social responsibility are related.

Green-Wilson J, Zeigler S, eds.
Learning to Lead in Physical Therapy (pp 193-213).
© 2020 Taylor & Francis Group.

Leadership Vignette

Richard Jackson, PT, OCS

I have never thought of myself as socially responsible, or even considered my activities as such. My choice of becoming a physical therapist originated from a conscious desire to help people. I think most physical therapists would say the same. Physical therapists have a natural inclination to help others, so by nature, we are socially responsible. Social responsibility can also mean service. Call it what you will—I have always enjoyed helping people. It makes me feel good. What better way to spend a day than to spend it helping others?

My wife, Anna, and I have always embraced the notion that when you find your place in this world, you should help others find theirs. The nature and extent of the help, of course, depend on personal resources and comfort zones. We made a conscious decision to instill service to others in our practice: everything from adopting families at Thanksgiving and Christmas, to taking collections in our offices of warm winter clothing for the homeless, to providing physical therapy services pro bono. These activities encourage our staff members to serve others and embed the idea of service in our company's culture. It takes a conscious effort on our part, and our staff members participate eagerly. We create the opportunity to serve, and we do not force anyone to participate. We make the connections and create the structure. Our patients participate as well. Everyone wins, especially those we serve—low-cost, high-impact.

In 2010, we decided to start an educational project in a developing country. Our purpose was, in part, to offer our clinical staff a personal and cultural experience to broaden their horizons. We decided to serve overseas, committed to it, and then looked for an opportunity. This decision really embedded service in our company culture.

Ultimately, we chose Africa because we understand the culture (I was a Peace Corps volunteer in Kenya in 1978), and we feel comfortable in that area of the world. Our Ethiopian venture started when one of our clinic directors, who had been born and raised in Ethiopia but educated in the United States, decided to return to his country to assist in raising the level of education in his homeland. We joined his mission, started an orthopedic residency program, and eventually developed a curriculum outline for a doctor of physical therapy program to be launched at Addis Ababa University. It was the first doctor of physical therapy program in Africa. This program led to connections that brought us to Kenya, where we have developed another orthopedic residency program.

Our African experience has changed lives—those of our staff, and those of our African students and citizens. We have changed the course of rehabilitation in 2 countries. This has had a profound impact on us as individuals, and has resulted in rich personal rewards. There is a deep satisfaction in giving others the opportunity to grow. Our staff members who come back from a trip universally report that they will never look at the world the same way again. They have developed lasting friendships and report that they feel personally transformed. Again, they gain a deep satisfaction by helping people in need through service.

You do not need to serve or exercise social responsibility in a developing country. Many opportunities exist in your own town, nearest city, county, or state. You can serve others wherever you are most comfortable; it costs nothing to give your time. However, if you are interested in creating a more global impact, there are monetary costs involved depending on where you want to begin your project and the nature of the project. If you are committed to leading by serving in the United States or abroad, the following steps will help:

- Decide to serve.
- Identify a need.

- Make connections; opportunity will come your way.
- Have the confidence that you can meet the need and it is in your comfort zone.
- Invest in the need.
- Be creative and work within the culture.

Regardless of what you decide, the rewards are enormous and your life will be enriched. If you are a practice owner, the idea of servant leadership will transform your staff and your company culture. You will receive far more than you give by seeing your staff grow and mature through service to others.

SOCIAL RESPONSIBILITY DEFINED

Individuals who are socially responsible behave in ways that are ethical and sensitive toward social, economic, cultural, and environmental issues. Socially responsible individuals embrace social responsibility as a lifestyle and contribute to socially responsible activities such as recycling, volunteering, donating, and mentoring.

Individual social responsibility means that each person within a community is engaged in some way. Engagement can be expressed as demonstrating an interest toward what is happening within a community, as well as active participation in solving some of the local or community's problems. Other examples of engagement include taking part in street or local neighborhood cleaning initiatives; organizing an event; or helping children (with or without parents) or elderly people.

Individuals who are socially responsible often put pressure on organizations to become more socially responsible. For example, many companies have integrated social responsibility into their business models by going "green," or by adopting practices such as recycling, buying local, and minimizing driving to be more supportive of the environment and for sustainability. Another common example of passive individual social responsibility supported through an organization is when a company establishes a system whereby individuals donate to a designated nonprofit organization such as United Way or to charities from a selected menu of options. Typically, this model deducts donations from an individual's paycheck on a predetermined schedule, and then the businesses forward the total monies collected to each organization. A small amount of effort is needed to orchestrate this type of giving program, and often modest revenues are allocated through this initiative. Sometimes organizations add a corporate matching gift effort. In this model, individuals donate, and the physical therapist practice or health care organization matches this donation, typically up to a specified dollar amount. Although this corporate-matching effort may raise more funds, it still requires minimal time or effort on the part of the employees or the executives of the organization.

Corporate social responsibility (CSR) refers to the commitment of business to contribute to sustainable economic development, working with employees, their families, the local community and society at large to improve their quality of life.[1] TOMS Shoes (www.toms.com) is an example of an organization that has integrated CSR into its core business model. TOMS Shoes was founded on the social mission of matching every pair of shoes purchased with a pair of new shoes for a child in need. In general, CSR requires businesses to develop a positive relationship with the society and environments in which they operate. According to the International Organization for Standardization, this relationship is "a critical factor in their ability to continue to operate effectively. It is also increasingly being used as a measure of their overall performance."[2(p8)] More and more, companies are experiencing pressure to be accountable to stakeholders including employees, consumers, suppliers, local communities, policymakers, and society-at-large, in addition to their ongoing obligation to shareholders.[2] When defined strategically, CSR therefore encompasses what companies do with their profits, as well as how they make them.[3]

The concept of CSR may be framed in different ways by different organizations within different countries. For example, some suggest that CSR in the United States aligns more closely to a philanthropic or charitable model. In this model of CSR, companies make profits, virtually unconstrained, except for fulfilling their duty to pay taxes, and then they may donate a specified share of the profits to humanitarian causes. Some argue that this approach to CSR may not seem totally clean because the company may receive tax benefits from giving. In contrast, some suggest that in Europe, CSR may be more sustainable because at the core, businesses fundamentally focus on operating in a socially responsible way, balanced by investing in situations and communities for concrete business reasons. In this way, social responsibility becomes an integral part of the wealth creation process and the vision and mission of the organization, and that even during tough economic times, organizations may still continue to practice CSR because it is so intertwined into the life of the business. In contrast, in the US philanthropic model, CSR may often be seen as peripheral to the core business, meaning that CSR may be the first item cut when the financial bottom line looks weak.

Social Justice: Understanding the Need for Social Responsibility in Health Care

Social justice, or fairness, involves the belief that everyone deserves equal economic, political, and social rights and opportunities. Therefore, a socially just society is based on the principles of equality and solidarity, understands and values human rights, and recognizes the dignity of every human being. When there is real or perceived injustice within our communities, individuals with a common ideology often come together, and social movements begin in which these groups of people try to achieve certain goals together.

Social justice should be central to health care. Consider the contemporary yet controversial topic of providing affordable access to health care to vulnerable populations such as seniors and individuals from low-income households. Also, consider the mediocre or poor performance of the US health care system in terms of managing chronic disease and community-based care.[4] Health care should be efficient, driven by evidence and current research, cost-effective, and offered to all citizens within the United States. Yet, people wonder if health care in this country is viewed as a right or a privilege. Can people accept the fact that vulnerable populations have a much higher mortality birth rate and earlier death rates in the United States? Questions arise as to whether society should bear the cost of health care for low-income families, or if leveraging consumer-driven health care would be a better choice in addressing this concern. Some believe that health care could be very simple: the well should take care of the sick.[4] Unfortunately, much of health care today is not sustainable, especially from a financial perspective. Verkerk et al define *sustainable health care* as a complex system interacting to restore, manage, and optimize human health, and working harmoniously with the human body and the non-human environment from an ecological base that is viable indefinitely from environmental, economic, and social perspectives.[5] Some argue that if waste in the current health care system were merely reduced, then excellent health care at a lower cost could be offered to all.[6]

A-HA! – YOUR OPINION

Should health care be a basic legal right for every individual in the United States, or is health care a privilege for those who earn it?

_____

Why do you think you feel this way?

_____

_____

Social Responsibility and the Physical Therapist

Social responsibility, in physical therapist practice, is the promotion of mutual trust between the profession and the larger public that necessitates responding to societal needs for health and wellness.[7] Without a doubt, social responsibility will play an essential role in helping physical therapists and physical therapist assistants pursue the new vision for the profession of physical therapy, as transforming society relies on the capacity of individual professionals to be responsible for the needs of societal members.

Activity 11-1: Individual Social Responsibility in Physical Therapy

Social responsibility is one of the 7 core values of professionalism the American Physical Therapy Association (APTA) has identified in physical therapy.[7] For this activity, visit http://www.apta.org/CoreValuesSelfAssessment/ProfessionalDuty/ and assess yourself on the behaviors identified in the APTA Core Values Self-Assessment.[8]

Social Responsibility in Physical Therapy: Satisfying the Need to Lead

Each individual within a physical therapist practice and the profession of physical therapy has an active role to play in achieving socially responsible obligations for society.

A socially responsible leader recognizes the virtues within others and encourages those within a community to use personal talents to contribute to the benefit of the whole. A socially responsible leader leads for the common good: the greatest possible good for the greatest possible number of individuals. Purtilo, in the 31st APTA Mary McMillan lecture in 2000, challenged all physical therapists to embark on a "period of social identity."[9] She emphasized that the moral foundation of a true professional is one who partners with a larger community of citizens. She encouraged those in the profession to reflect on who they are—individually as professionals, and collectively as a profession—and to identify what responsibilities they must accept to truly be recognized as professionals. As physical therapy moved to a profession with education at the clinical doctoral level, she encouraged practitioners to explore and accept societal obligations consistent with the profession's higher aspirations.[9]

A-HA! – SOCIALLY RESPONSIBLE LEADERS

Many of the action-oriented verbs describing the behaviors of social responsibility (Activity 11-1) included the words *advocate*, *promote*, and *participate*.

Take a few moments to identify specific behaviors you would expect to see a physical therapist demonstrate as a socially responsible leader who:

- Advocates _____

- Promotes _____

- Participates _____

Bottom Line!

"Until the great mass of the people shall be filled with the sense of responsibility for each other's welfare, social justice can never be attained." – Helen Keller, American author, political activist, and lecturer

LEADERSHIP STYLES OF THE SOCIALLY RESPONSIBLE

In their book, *Leading With Soul*, Bolman and Deal acknowledge that leadership is giving; the gift of leaders is to give themselves to a cause or a vision that is greater than themselves.[10] Leadership is a journey of interconnectedness among values such as love, significance, power, and authorship for a common good.[10] Leadership from this lens moves individuals from being self-centered to being other-centered (ie, community). Know that the roles as leaders in for-profit or nonprofit businesses reach beyond the bottom line. Such decisions may be described from the utilitarian (useful) ethical perspective in which people make decisions based on the greatest good, or from the communitarian (collective) perspective in which value within a community is more important than personal interests and self-recognition. In either case, actions illustrate how important community is to a leader and decision-maker.

Recall that in Chapter 3, classic and contemporary leadership styles were introduced, as well as the importance of influencing others as leaders, behaviors of effective and ineffective leadership styles, and the style of followership. Recall that leadership is about behaviors; in this way, it is meaningful to translate theories of leadership into behaviors or styles of leadership. Style is a distinct way of expressing or conducting oneself; it is a pattern of behavior. Typically, the style used by individuals will reflect their beliefs, values, mindsets, passions, and preferences, as well as any organizational systems' culture and norms that encourage some styles and discourage others. Converting leadership theories into leadership styles helps define a range of observable behaviors or approaches that can be used by individuals interested in becoming more effective as leaders.

In this chapter, the discussion of leadership styles will be expanded by examining 2 styles that seem to emulate characteristics of leaders who are socially responsible in their approach to leadership. Specifically, the leadership styles of servant leaders and "Level 5 Leaders" will be examined.[11-13]

The Style of the Servant Leader

Recall that you were introduced to servant leaders in Chapter 3. Servant leadership is less about *what* these leaders actually do and more about *why* these leaders do what they do. Servant leaders fundamentally look at leadership as an act of service, and they focus primarily on the needs of others rather than how others can serve or follow them.[13] In contrast, leaders who are more self-serving in their approach to leadership spend most of their time protecting their own interests and status, fear losing their power, and do not invest time mentoring others.[12] Frederick Douglass, Harriet Tubman, and Mahatma Gandhi are 3 famous examples of servant leaders; a brief description of these servant leaders is provided in Box 11-1.

The servant leader's behavior is driven by a particular set of principles, values, passions, and beliefs.[14] The style of the servant leader is characterized by empathy, listening, forward-thinking, imagination, stewardship, the ethical use of power and empowerment, and community-building.[13] Servant leaders are collaborative and cooperative. Essentially, they spend much of their time and energy supporting the growth, recognition, and success of their followers. They assume responsibility for their followers, put their followers' well-being before tasks or goals, and connect with their followers in a variety of ways so that, ultimately, their followers achieve, flourish, and improve. Servant leadership is a means for transforming hearts, heads, hands, and habits to serve others, and loyalty, trust, and productivity result within these servant leader-follower relationships.[12]

A-HA! – SERVANT LEADERSHIP AND YOU

Servant leadership begins first with a serving heart rather than a self-serving ambition; this means that the servant leader first considers the benefits and consequences for those they lead, rather than the benefits to the servant leader.[12]

Box 11-1

FAMOUS SERVANT LEADERS

- **Frederick Douglass**, a former slave and a well-known and active leader of the abolitionist movement, was the first black citizen to hold a high US government rank. Douglass gained support through his persuasive oratory and insightful writings about antislavery; he also actively supported women's suffrage.

- **Harriet Tubman** escaped slavery to become a leading abolitionist. She led hundreds of enslaved people to freedom along the route of the Underground Railroad.

- **Mahatma Gandhi**, considered the father of the Indian independence movement, spent 20 years in South Africa working to fight discrimination. While in India, he spent his remaining years working diligently to both remove British rule from India as well as to better the lives of India's poorest classes.

When was the last time you feel you demonstrated servant leadership?

_____

_____

_____

What were the aspects of this style of leadership that you feel you demonstrated most?

_____

_____

_____

How do you see servant leadership as a style most effective for socially responsible leaders?

_____

_____

_____

The Style of the Humble Leader With Professional Will: Level 5 Leadership

Collins, in his book, *Good to Great*, highlighted Level 5 Leaders as having the type of executive or formal leadership required for transforming a good company into a great one.[11] Collins distinguished 5 levels of leaders, each level appropriate in certain situations (Figure 11-1).[11]

In Collins' model, *Level 1 Leaders*, described as "Highly Capable Individuals," make useful contributions through talent, competency, and diligent work. *Level 2 Leaders* are seen as the "Contributing Team Members" because they influence the achievement of group objectives positively and work effectively with others in group situations. *Level 3 Leaders*, or "Competent Managers," are successful at organizing people and resources in effectively and efficiently achieving established goals and objectives. *Level 4 Leaders*, characterized as the "Effective Leaders," transform energy and commitments

Figure 11-1. The style of the humble leader with professional will—Level 5 Leadership. (Reprinted with permission from Collins J. *Good to Great*. New York, NY: HarperCollins Publishers, Inc.; 2001:20.)

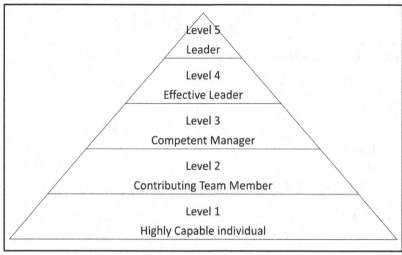

in pursuit of a compelling vision, and stimulate high performance from the group and its members. Finally, *Level 5 Leaders* possess all of the characteristics identified in the other 4 levels of leadership, plus they merge "extreme personal humility with extraordinary professional will."[11(p13)]

Essentially, Level 5 Leaders are at the top of this framework or hierarchy of leadership capabilities. Abraham Lincoln is considered an example of a Level 5 Leader in that he did not let his ego get in the way of his ambition to create a lasting, great nation. Individuals do not need to proceed sequentially through each level of this leadership framework to reach the top levels, but to be considered a Level 5 Leader, individuals need to possess the capabilities of the other 4 levels plus the unique characteristics needed at Level 5.[11]

A Level 5 Leader is described as someone who is not boastful or arrogant, but is modest and humble. These leaders produce tremendous results but shun public recognition. They use "we" language, not "I" language. For example, these leaders may describe the work that "we did," not the work that "I did as the leader," because they understand the importance of a team in achieving outstanding results. Level 5 Leaders help others and show respect toward others. Level 5 Leaders are humble, and their humility helps them be effective learners because they know they do not know everything and need to be open-minded enough to seek out new information. It is important to highlight that when Level 5 Leaders and other individuals approach situations from a perspective of humility, possibilities such as curiosity and open-mindedness open up within teams; openness discourages leaders from adopting a certain position to protect their own points of view.[15]

Activity 11-2: Developing Humility

Humility may help facilitate your self-development; being humble allows you to be more honest with yourself. Humility may also help you improve your relationships.[11,15] Table 11-1 offers a few ways for you to develop and practice humility. Self-assess using this list, and ask others to assess you as well.

Bottom Line!

Socially responsible leaders step back, encourage others, and are supportive as others gain visibility. Socially responsible leaders focus on helping others benefit and gain value.

TABLE 11-1. HUMILITY SELF-ASSESSMENT	
HUMILITY CHARACTERISTIC	**SELF OR OTHER RATING** *0 = Never* *1 = Sometimes* *2 = Often* *3 = Always*
You behave humbly. Whenever your team succeeds, you make sure that team members get the credit for their hard work.	
You catch yourself from overpreaching or coaching without permission. You consider whether you are trying to impose your point of view before actually doing so.	
You stop talking and allow other people to talk.	
You practice saying, "You're right."	
You are willing to share your weaknesses with people you trust. You acknowledge your limitations.	
You practice gentleness and kindness; speak well of others; and respond to other's attacks, actions, and criticisms with gentleness, patience, and respect. You do not react negatively or defensively.	
You are open to and receive feedback from others graciously, and you look for a kernel of truth in what people tell you, even if it comes from a debatable source.	

SOCIAL ENTREPRENEURSHIP

Social entrepreneurs identify and solve social problems. They act as change agents for society, seizing opportunities that are often overlooked, to improve systems, disseminate new and innovative approaches, and advance sustainable solutions that create social value. Social entrepreneurship applies the principles of entrepreneurship to organize, create, and manage social undertakings to achieve a desired social change. In general, successful entrepreneurs or entrepreneurial leaders exhibit certain attitudes and behaviors organized around 6 dominant themes (Table 11-2).[16]

Note that leadership is one of the top 6 characteristics of entrepreneurs, and recall from Chapter 9 that change requires leadership. Even though social entrepreneurs primarily seek to produce social rather than monetary value, they still know the importance of accessing resources, including monies and key stakeholders, to be successful in leading any sustainable change.

There are many opportunities for physical therapists to lead as socially responsible leaders and as social entrepreneurs. Since 2006, Brad Thuringer, a physical therapist assistant and Academic Coordinator of Clinical Education for the Physical Therapist Assistant Program at Lake Area Technical Institute in Watertown, South Dakota, has engaged the physical therapy community from across the United States in an annual outreach effort for Shoes4Kids (Figure 11-2). Shoes4Kids is focused on serving underprivileged and underserved children and their families by providing them with new, brand name athletic shoes. As a result of Thuringer's social entrepreneurial efforts and the response from the physical therapy community, Shoes4Kids has provided more than 15,000 pairs of shoes and multitudes of socks to underprivileged families in the United States.

TABLE 11-2. DESIRABLE AND ACQUIRABLE ATTITUDES AND BEHAVIORS OF SUCCESSFUL ENTREPRENEURS	
THEMES	**BEHAVIOR OR ATTITUDE**
Commitment and determination	Tenacious and decisive, able to commit and recommit quickly
	Persistent in solving problems, disciplined
	Immersed
Leadership	Self-starter with high standards, but not a perfectionist
	Honest and reliable; builds trust; practices fairness
	Team builder; inspires others
Opportunity obsession	Market-driven
	Obsessed with value-creation and enhancement
Tolerance of risk, ambiguity, and uncertainty	Calculated risk-taker
	Risk-minimizer
	Tolerates uncertainty and lack of structure
Creativity, self-reliance, and adaptability	Nonconventional; open-minded, lateral thinker
	Restless with the status quo
	No fear of failure
Motivation to excel	Drive to achieve and grow
	Low need for status and power
	Aware of weaknesses and strengths
Reprinted with permission from Timmons JA, Spinelli S. *New Venture Creation, Entrepreneurship for the 21st Century.* New York, NY: McGraw-Hill Irwin; 2007:8.	

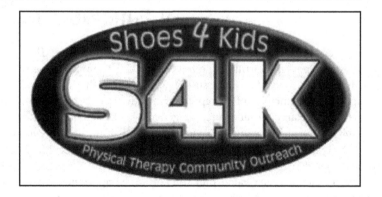

Figure 11-2. Shoes4Kids Logo.

As the profession of physical therapy continues to earn its autonomy as it evolves within the health care industry, it becomes even more apparent that collectively, physical therapists can assume leadership roles at the societal level. Sandstrom describes professional autonomy as "a social contract based on public trust in an occupation to meet a significant social need and to preserve individual autonomy."[17(p98)] Moreover, continuous change within health care presents evolving opportunities for physical therapists as professionals to renegotiate their contract with society.[18] It is critical that physical therapists recognize their professional autonomy as a social contract based on the public's trust and service to meet the health needs of people who are experiencing disablement to maintain their individual autonomy.[17] Then, as a profession, they need to continue to develop and demonstrate behaviors of social responsibility, leadership, and professionalism to earn and retain society's trust. S. M. R. Covey, in his book, *The SPEED of TRUST*, claims that "the overriding principle of societal trust is contribution. It's the intent to create value instead of destroy it, to give back instead of take. More people are realizing how important contribution and the causes it inspires, are to a healthy society."[19(p275)]

A-HA! – TRUST IN SELF AND TRUST IN OTHERS

Notice how trust comes up again and again in this book. In Chapter 2, the focus was on self-trust; in Chapter 6, the need was for development of trust for effective teamwork; and in this chapter, trust with society is vital to preserving the essence of the profession of physical therapy. Establishing, maintaining, and renewing trust at all levels are foundational skills for those learning to lead.

Review your trust self-assessment from Table 2-3 in Chapter 2. Then, review your A-Ha! – Trust in Others responses from Chapter 6 on page 108.

How do ensuring self-trust and building the trust of others help in promoting societal trust?

_____

_____

Provide at least 3 examples of how you can use social responsibility behaviors to build and renew societal trust in the profession of physical therapy.

_____

_____

_____

●────────────────

Bottom Line!

Social entrepreneurs identify and solve societal problems with the strong sense of social responsibility. Effective entrepreneurial leaders pay particular attention to the contract between themselves and society, focusing on the establishment and maintenance of trust.

SOCIAL CONSCIOUSNESS: VOLUNTEERISM AND SERVICE

Leaders with soul and a social conscience who appreciate the social responsibility of their role develop lives that have meaning, purpose, and joy, and contribute to something that is much greater than they are—they contribute to the community.[10] Leaders with social conscience value how their business or organization impacts their local, regional, or international community. Often organizations encourage employees to volunteer in their community. Numerous US nonprofit organizations exist because of volunteerism. Organizations may expect and encourage employees to volunteer in areas in which each individual is passionate, or these companies may select specific opportunities in which employee can participate as a group, either during the week or on a weekend. Sometimes, individuals may be allotted a few (ie, 1 to 5) paid "mission days" each year within their employee benefit package to participate as volunteers offering service for the day in activities that support nonprofit organizations or social programs. These models engage individuals in actual service projects while involving the employer, who pays the individuals typically their usual pay to participate in this service effort. In this way, the individuals do not lose income, and the company demonstrates efforts to promote social responsibility. Alternatively, an employer may offer to split the cost of donated services with the employees, so half the time spent is unpaid.

It is important to clarify that volunteering is a steppingstone to raising social awareness; however, it lacks the critical piece needed to help people truly develop a sense of social consciousness and sustainable social responsibility. For example, when physical therapists offer health screens for free or at a significantly reduced cost, some classify this activity as public relations, while others refer to it as being socially responsible. When physical therapists participate in these volunteer activities and use these events primarily for public relations or promotion, then the intent behind their participation seems to be more focused on increasing their presence and recognition in the community vs participating to contribute to the betterment of a particular group or community.

In contrast to volunteerism, providing pro bono services as physical therapists and providing physical therapy services to underserved and underrepresented populations are common ways for serving communities as socially responsible leaders. In the APTA's *Physical Therapist Code of Ethics*, pro bono services are explicitly noted as exemplar activities to demonstrate social responsibility. Many law firms incorporate this type of service as well by expecting lawyers within the practice to offer a certain amount of pro bono services per year. This represents true service, as the practicing lawyers typically do not get paid to provide for such services, but rather donate their personal time. Typically, they reach out to individuals or nonprofit organizations that are unable to secure legal help because of the cost. Many jurisdictions solicit pro bono legal service from the legal community, on a rotating basis, for individuals within their community who meet certain socioeconomic or other hardship levels.

Understanding the intent behind volunteering and service is foundational in distinguishing these actions. Specifically, volunteering may be viewed as an act of charity, whereas service may be viewed as an opportunity for relationship-building within the community. Therefore, it is critical for socially responsible leaders to clearly articulate their expectations, be purposeful in action, and share their intent explicitly with their followers and the people with whom they are engaging.

A-HA! – SOCIAL CONSCIOUSNESS AND INTENTION

Think about an experience in which you volunteered, and reflect upon the intent or the reasons why you took this action.

_____

_____

_____

Reflect upon what you (as an individual and/or as an organization/group) were hoping to gain from the experience. In other words, were you volunteering for business reasons (ie, promotion and publicity) or for altruistic or socially responsible reasons?

_____

_____

_____

Bottom Line!

Being aware of your intentions when engaging with the public and society at large is a key step toward representing yourself and your profession responsibly. Effective leaders have a healthy sense of social consciousness and are able to articulate intentions clearly and purposefully.

Social Responsibility: Leadership Through Advocacy

As mentioned earlier in this chapter, advocacy is an important component of social responsibility. For instance, physical therapists and physical therapist assistants often advocate for those with disabilities, for those without access to health care services, and for those entering the profession carrying a lot of debt that may interfere with their ability to make socially responsible decisions. Therefore, it is essential for physical therapists to consider their ongoing roles as advocates and subsequent opportunities for advocacy within the everchanging health care environment.

Advocacy means action; it is a process used to influence decision making within political, economic, and/or social systems, including public policy and resource-allocation decisions. Advocacy efforts may range from more passive to more active efforts within physical therapist practice. Examples of passive advocacy may include avoiding socially harmful acts or donating money to support socially responsible activities, efforts, and/or programs that benefit those whom are served. More active approaches to advocacy may include participation in activities that advance social goals such as securing funding to support research efforts in health care or promoting employment laws that advance the rights of employees in business practices.

Activity 11-3: Planning to Advocate

When you are planning to advocate for your patients/clients, industry, profession, community, or team, consider when your advocacy may be most effective. In other words, use your time wisely. Remember that you have unique knowledge about a specific field or topic, and others depend on you for sharing this information. How you convey this information will be important. For this activity, use the following steps and plan out an action that you can take to advocate for patients, the community, or the profession.

Step 1: Educate yourself about the situation or scenario for which you want to advocate so you can be prepared and organized. What topic interests you?

_____

Step 2: Build allies in advance. Build diverse networks of support. Which people do you need on your team, and why?

_____

_____

_____

Step 3: Learn about your legislators (decision makers) and other key stakeholders in advance. On what committees do they serve? What are their positions on specific issues? What are their priorities? Determine ways to capture their attention; determine the hook or the compelling story.

_____

_____

_____

Step 4: Establish and maintain relationships. Keep good notes and follow up consistently on everything. Plan for follow up on your efforts, and list 1 to 2 ways you will do that.

_____

_____

_____

Leadership and Advocacy Styles

Advocacy is practiced for different reasons, and different situations require different styles or approaches. Essentially, advocates can provide self-advocacy, group advocacy, peer advocacy, or legal advocacy, as described here:

- *Self-advocacy* occurs when individuals speak up for themselves to express their own needs and represent their own interests.
- *Group advocacy* occurs when individuals work together to represent their shared interests or goals and/or seek development or change in services.
- *Peer advocacy* may occur when one individual feels more courageous to speak up for other individuals who share the same issues, experiences, difficulties, or discrimination.
- *Legal advocacy* means representation by legally qualified advocates, usually attorneys.

In any form, advocacy requires a passion for the issues and the drive to make a change. Therefore, leaders as advocates may need to develop specific skills to strengthen their ability to advocate effectively. Key skills and qualities needed for effective advocacy may include assertiveness, the ability to craft a well-defined message or vision, strong networking skills to recruit support from community members, communication skills to convey a compelling and confident message, effective listening skills to sincerely hear and understand all perspectives, and a strong commitment to persevere regardless of the challenges. Successful advocacy also requires leaders to be prepared, be organized, and understand how the system works. It may be useful in advance to anticipate the range of possible perspectives or wants related to a potentially controversial issue, and to anticipate the wants and possible responses before the negotiation begins. As part of the preparatory process, it may also be helpful for advocates to be clear about the role in which they serve: are they facilitators? coordinators? protectors? Clarifying the advocacy goal is as important as stating the intention of social consciousness efforts. For instance, is the ultimate goal a mutual win-win, or will the outcome most likely be a win-lose? All these factors may impact the style or approach used by leaders to advocacy initiatives.

Activity 11-4: Advocacy Is About the Messaging

Have you considered the best ways to get your message across and to gain attention for your cause? To further develop your skills in leading for change, take a moment to consider the following ideas in crafting your message(s):

- Practice professional assertiveness. Being assertive does not mean you have to be aggressive; preparation will help you have the confidence to state your situation clearly, succinctly, and knowledgeably.
- Create effective hooks. What message will get their attention? Hooks may need to change depending on the audience.
- Practice effective interviewing skills. Create 2-way dialogue rather than a monologue.
- Share needs and successes with peers who can give you honest and strategic feedback.
- End every conversation with a request (the "ask") and with the goal of getting a commitment. Consider making a request that provides an opportunity for follow-up.
- Guarantee the commitment. Follow through with your request. Some follow-up actions may include providing resources, offering clarification, and referring people to experts if you do not have the answers.
- Be sure to thank them for their time and thank them again if/when they support you.

Now, take your idea from Activity 11-3, and create your message script for your advocacy topic.

_____

_____

_____

_____

_____

_____

_____

_____

_____

_____

_____

_____

_____

Bottom Line!

True leaders see their role as a vocation; it is a lifestyle that encourages others to join their movement.[20,21]

Case Study: Social Responsibility and Leadership

As you read these 2 stories, consider the following questions:

1. When did they start becoming more socially responsible as physical therapists, and why? How and when did they start, and what happened when they started being more socially responsible?
2. How did being socially responsible physical therapists transform them, as well as others around them?
3. How do they define *social responsibility*? Why do they feel that social responsibility is important for physical therapists?
4. In their opinions, what challenges do we face in becoming more socially responsible as a profession? What benefits can we gain?
5. In their opinions, what impact can one socially responsible person make?
6. What has been the biggest challenge for them—as individual personal leaders—in leading (or working with) diverse groups? Why was this difficult?
   > How did they overcome this challenge? What did they do differently? What did they learn?
7. What wisdom did they share for individuals such as you in developing personal leadership skills and the ability to lead (work within) diverse groups effectively?
8. What process have they used to discover their core values? How important are their core values in guiding them as leaders?
9. What are they most passionate about as leaders in physical therapy?
10. What are their leadership strengths, and how do they use their strengths?
11. How important is passion for leadership?
12. How important is authenticity in being effective as a leader?
13. In their opinion, what leadership skills do we need to develop and have to be more socially responsible as health care professionals?

Efosa L. Guobadia, DPT

A turning point for me in the journey of social awareness and my responsibility to those around me was from my time as a student at the University of Scranton. The school's Jesuit tradition encouraged students to be "men and women for others." Along with that encouragement, you were required to serve actively in your community in ways that you felt called, and in ways that you discerned would benefit others. Through those efforts, whether you expected it or not, and sought it or not, a transformation happened. You felt the full bidirectionality that permeates through every moment of serving. In one direction, you are personally fulfilled through grace, and in the other direction, you are provided the privilege to fulfill others through compassion.

That time in my life has catalyzed so much of what has come after. Serving and being socially responsible to my environment and fellow community members is worthy to do as well as worth doing. It now represents so much of my existence and what I believe in. A life of service is a life in full. We all have a heart and, thus, we can all do it. The world needs it.

Being socially responsible transcends any hat that you may have on at the moment. Being socially responsible is a mindset that needs to be curated both daily and intentionally, no matter where or with whom you find yourself. The beautiful thing about being socially responsible is that the different hats that we wear in life allow for different forms of social responsibility to manifest themselves. Caring for, listening to, and taking time with my patient in clinics in the United States has given me the strength to share my food with those who were hungry in countries abroad. The same is true in reverse. When we lead by serving, those examples send positive ripples that can lead to transformation in others.

To be socially responsible to your community and those in it is to be intentional and responsible in an effort to effectuate positive change in the life of one or many. Ideally, your efforts are along a sustainable continuum and bereft of jingoistic or patronizing behaviors. Physical therapists are equipped with the beautiful tools that are our hands and hearts and words. With those tools, we can go anywhere and be helpful to many. That capacity for affecting others gives us great responsibility, and the assuming of and leaning into that responsibility can give us great capacity to positively affect others.

The profession of physical therapy is full of so many who are compassionate and who perform socially responsible acts in micro and macro ways each day, within the clinic and beyond the clinic walls. There is an opportunity for us to perform and display these efforts in a more connected way in the communities where we reside and as a profession as a whole. When these efforts are more salient, we will be one of the professions that the country and the world looks to when pain points arise in our society, within the health care realm and without. I believe that will push us to be our best. I believe we will be ready.

One act of good can change the world. I call it *exponential love*. By helping one person's life be better, you positively affect the family unit and overall ecosystem. When you positively affect the person's ecosystem, that, in turn, betters the community. Better communities lead to a better world. The hope is that these positive acts, no matter at what level they start, are happening many times and continuously in communities all around the globe. Those ripples of good lead to an unstoppable wave of change.

Over the years, I have pushed myself to be more aware of how best to cultivate the right pace for the group with whom I am working. The pace is predicated on needs of the group's objective multiplied to the makeup and needs of the group. That takes understanding each member individually and the group as a whole; solidifying group dynamics; coming together as soon as possible; getting everyone in alignment; seeing the same vision; and helping them discern how they can all contribute to its pursuit. I have also found that when you empower others, they will do empowering things. Ultimately, communication and action are how you get things done.

Communication is paramount. If you can talk about things, you can work through almost anything. This includes the things that you may need to fix or play defense on, as well as for positive opportunities that arise and that allow you to go on offense. Being a great communicator and fostering open communication by everyone on the team allows the group to move, as Covey titled his book, at *The SPEED of TRUST*.[19]

This quote from Ronald Reagan resonates: "The greatest leader is not necessarily the one who does the greatest things. He is the one that gets the people to do the greatest things."

Leaders who enable and empower the happening of great work, near and far from them, give the organization its best chance to succeed.

Meditation, prayer, and reflection have been part of the process that has shaped my core values. I start with the foundation of what my non-negotiables are, and what I want to be able to measure my actions and words by. Those concretes form the foundation of my values. As I mature and grow, so do they. My core values are my everything. They are my North Star when I need guidance. They are my dynamic compass that helps me navigate both the clear path as well as the occluded one.

I am most passionate about the potential within each student, clinician, and general participant of the profession of physical therapy. Our profession attracts special people, and , in turn, those people are capable of special things. I want to be part of the unleashing of the transformative change that is currently happening and continues to happen through this passionate critical mass. What is brewing and is possible—that fires me up each and every day.

What I try to be most intentional with is connecting with each person in the group in a personal and precise way, and empowering them to connect to the whole group and the group's objective in ways that are unique to them. When the whole team is working together, it leads to a glorious symphony.

Passion multiplied by purpose is important for both leadership and life. Purpose is that constant rock that is steady against the waves of time and circumstances. Passion is a fuel that allows you to inspire others and to rise up along with the team to challenges and opportunities. When the whole team is passionate about the unifying objectives and fundamental value that you all are collectively trying to provide, obstacles disappear, and opportunities and the way forward arise.

Being genuine and authentic is integral to being a long-term leader because your authentic self and style are what you know how to do best, and what are most real. In the challenging situations especially, your authentic self will rise high and be seen. In those situations, it is best that your team is not wholly surprised. The skill to collaborate with others needs to be continuously cultivated. In that collaboration, be sure that the results are additive or multiplicative, as opposed to subtractive. Diversity can lead to dynamicity, and when things get dynamic, anything is possible, and everything can change.

Joshua D'Angelo, PT, DPT

As physical therapists, athletes, and students, many of us have been in situations of great opportunity or great need. It might be the chance to compete for a championship, the opportunity to start a new and innovative initiative, or the demand of solving a complex problem. Each of these moments brings questions as we strive for success. How can we inspire and uplift our team to compete at our highest level? How can we build something brand new to make our program better and more effective than ever before? How can we draw out the unique knowledge and experience of each team member to find a solution collaboratively? As we dive into each question, a pattern quickly emerges: the stronger and more empowered each team member is, the more likely we are to succeed.

Throughout high school, college, graduate school, and beyond, I kept the concept of an empowered team at the forefront of my mind and consistently asked how I could better serve those around me. The more I focused on giving to, encouraging, and inspiring others, the more that others began to look at me as a leader. The skillsets I developed as a servant leader directly impact my ability to successfully treat patients as a health care provider.

By the nature of our oaths, intents, and education as physical therapists, we are obligated to put the interests of our patients ahead of our own. In exchange for our interest in using our education to help, our patients will give their trust to us. What we do with their trust—the effort we put into helping and healing, the dedication we demonstrate to their improvement, and how we advocate for their health—will determine our success as socially responsible physical therapists.

During my first service trip to Guatemala, we had a break from treatment in the middle of the day. I went out back behind our clinic, and found a group of children playing soccer. The field was primarily dirt with a sporadic patch of grass. Some kids had shoes, and some did not, but all had the same big smile. Watching them run, jump, laugh, and play, I realized that these children were no different than the children who were running, jumping, laughing, and playing in the United States; I realized that regardless of language, culture, socioeconomic status, we all have similar desires: to move better so that we can do the things we love, to spend time with our family and friends, and to contribute to our communities. In those moments, I saw a sense of common humanity and a sense of common purpose that unites different corners of the world.

Service has often provided me with moments of transformation, growth, and meaning, and I have been fortunate to witness that transformation in others as well. When working with fellow clinicians and students, we often see individuals who begin treating with some hesitation, unsure about their abilities to provide great care in an unfamiliar environment, with a different culture, and a language barrier. Yet, over the course of a few hours or a few days, they are empowered by their skillset and the appreciation of those to whom they give. They realize the power they have in their hearts, hands, and minds to change and improve someone's life, regardless of their background, language, ethnicity, or culture. As they serve, hesitation turns into excitement, and uncertainty becomes confidence, knowledge, and cultural awareness.

Social responsibility, to me, is the obligation to give back to a society that has offered me so much—the opportunity for a safe childhood, with a great education, with the support of family and friends, and the resources needed to succeed. While I had to work hard to learn, grow, and achieve results, there is no way my success would have been possible without such a strong infrastructure underneath me and solid support behind me. Social responsibility means humbly recognizing all that contributed to your success and having the desire to make the infrastructure and support systems stronger for those around you and those who come after you.

As physical therapists, we have the unique ability to strengthen the societal infrastructure and support systems that help our patients succeed. In the United States and elsewhere, the stark reality is that many people need, but are not typically afforded, the opportunity to receive our services. Given our unique knowledge base, we have the potential to educate and weave a stronger fabric of health care within our society, helping others move better so they can live healthier and more fulfilling lives.

While our health care environment is changing rapidly and we live in a society where public discourse is often volatile, we have a profession that at its best is empathetic, compassionate, and effective. We have the opportunity to lead by example in taking quality care of our community members, regardless of the outside environment. It is the leaders who step up at times of challenge and confusion who are able to set the tone, expectations, and standards of care for the future.

A single person's voice can change the trajectory of a program, initiative, organization, and more. During my time at The George Washington University doctor of physical therapy program, one individual suggested we create a community service challenge for our program. Collectively, we decided to pursue the initiative, and in 2012, we launched our first Community Service Challenge. During the semester, we challenged our students and faculty to accumulate more than 1000 hours of community service. Through working with health fairs, pro bono clinics, a baseball team composed of individuals with disabilities, and much more, the program achieved its goal. The challenge became an annual tradition that lasted for years. What was once a single passionate voice turned into 1000 hours of service, and thousands more thereafter. A single socially responsible person has the potential to impact and change the lives of not only those who surround the person, but also the lives of an entire community.

I have been fortunate in my career to be surrounded by many passionate and talented leaders, with many great ideas. One of the challenges and unique opportunities I have faced has been uniting a diverse set of ideas to create the foundation for acting in a unified direction. As alignment is built, having motivated people all working toward the same mission and vision in a united fashion is a powerful combination. The team will grow together, learn together, and, with a bit of persistence and grit, ultimately succeed together.

Getting to know your teammates, and learning about their motivations, values, and goals, will enable you to develop trusting relationships with them. Trust is paramount in any team that is dedicated to the pursuit of a shared vision. One must communicate clearly, effectively, and efficiently to ensure the whole team remains on the same page and continues to work with inspiration and cohesion. It can take candor, maturity, and perseverance to ensure you are having the difficult and honest conversations that lead to progress.

On the personal leadership front, take the time to understand fully why you want to be influencing through leadership and what motivates you to lead. Then, craft and hone your ability to listen. When listening, intentionally observe, reflect on, and appreciate the thoughts and opinions that a diverse group can bring to the table. The differing perspectives will often lead to new and unique solutions that the group may have not considered before.

In Robert F. Kennedy's Day of Affirmation speech, he cites Archimedes, "...give me a place to stand, and I will move the earth." Leadership is a platform you stand on. It is a chance to leave a positive impact upon the world. Leadership is not centered on the concept of doing something for ourselves, but on creating meaningful change that will improve life for those around us. Physical therapy is a platform—a platform that has the potential to move the earth.

The process of discovering my core values has been 2-fold: looking internally and looking externally. First, I have taken time to reflect, ask myself why I am pursuing a course of action, and ensure that I am on a track I believe is fulfilling. Second, I have looked externally to leaders who resonate with me. When I find leaders I naturally gravitate toward, I take the time to listen to their speeches, read their books, converse with them when possible, and reflect upon what they are saying and why they are saying it. Many of the most charismatic, effective, and transformative leaders are guided by a strong set of principles. Their words and wisdom help influence my reflections and help me better understand my core values. Core values are, or should be, the most important factor in decision making. They are at the foundation of your team culture and should drive action. They are the core that all of your discussion and strategy center around—that is why they are called your "core" values.

The concept and belief in servant leadership—the fact that a leader's role is to make things better not for themselves, but for those around them—drives and centers my efforts. Too often, we focus ourselves upon what drives the most profit, how we can see the most patients, or how we can promote ourselves into a higher role. Yet, we forget why we went into this profession in the first place: to take great quality care of our patients, friends, family, and community. The central focus on how we can make life better both for our patients and for our professional colleagues is what fires me up on a daily basis.

Communication, consistency, and leading by example are at the center of my leadership philosophy. Clarity of communication helps empower your fellow teammates. Consistency in responsiveness and decision making enables others to trust you. Leading by example sets expectations and culture within the organization.

Candidly, I do not think passion for leadership is important to be a successful leader; rather, more important is a passion for an issue or problem that you are trying to solve. It is the passion for the idea that will keep driving you forward and motivating you to persevere. When others see your passion, it will be infectious and help the movement grow.

Authenticity enables trust, consistency, and understanding; authenticity centers us around our core values and provides transparent rationale for decisions. Without authenticity, we run the risk of being inconsistent, making decisions with differing rationales, and changing values, thereby creating a challenging environment for a team. However, with authenticity, our team can trust that a leader will be making decisions consistent with his or her core values based on what is in the best interest for the people and the success of the organization.

We must continue to put empathy and compassion at the forefront of all that we do as a profession. When we seek to understand and fully immerse ourselves in the perspectives of someone else, it enables trust, strong communication, and the opportunity to create a shared vision for the future. Whether you are working one-on-one with a patient, on a team, or within a large organization, you are a leader and have a platform on which you stand. With shared vision and a passion for solving complex problems, we can grow, make sustainable change, and create the best world we can imagine.

CHAPTER KEY WORDS

Social Responsibility, Social Justice, Social Entrepreneurship, Advocacy, Individual Social Responsibility, Corporate Social Responsibility, Social Conscience, Self-Advocacy, Peer Advocacy, Group Advocacy, Legal Advocacy

REFERENCES

1. Tonello M. *The Business Case for Corporate Social Responsibility: A Review of Concepts, Research and Practice.* https://corpgov.law.harvard.edu/2011/06/26/the-business-case-for-corporate-social-responsibility. Accessed March 25, 2020.

2. International Organization for Standardization. *Social Responsibility-ISO 26000.* http://www.iso.org/sr. Accessed November 2, 2018.

3. Harvard Kennedy School. *Corporate Social Responsibility Initiative.* https://www.hks.harvard.edu/centers/mrcbg/programs/cri. Accessed March 25, 2020.

4. Paul Farmer's Vision for Health. *News.* https://www.wgbh.org/news/post/paul-farmers-vision-health. Published May 17, 2013. Accessed October 10, 2018.

5. Verkerck MJ, DeLeede J, Nijhof AHJ. From responsible management to responsible organizations. *Bus Soc Rev.* 2001;106(4):353-378.

6.   Reid TR. *The Healing of America: A Global Quest for Better, Cheaper, and Fairer Health Care*. London, UK: Penguin; 2010.

7.   American Physical Therapy Association. *Professionalism in Physical Therapy: Core Values*. http://www.apta.org/ Professionalism. Accessed March 21, 2020.

8.   APTA Core Values Self-Assessment: Improving Professional Duty. http://www.apta.org/CoreValuesSelfAssessment/ ProfessionalDuty. Accessed October 10, 2018.

9.   Purtilo RB. A time to harvest, a time to sow: ethics for a shifting landscape. *Phys Ther*. 2000;80(11):1112.

10. Bolman LG, Deal TE. *Leading With Soul: An Uncommon Journey of Spirit*. Rev. 3rd ed. San Francisco, CA: Jossey-Bass; 2011.

11. Collins JC. *Good to Great: Why Some Companies Make the Leap... and Others Don't*. 1st ed. New York, NY: HarperBusiness; 2001.

12. Blanchard K. *Servant Leader*. Nashville, TN: Thomas Nelson; 2003.

13. What is Servant Leadership? *Greenleaf Cent Servant Leadership*. https://www.greenleaf.org/what-is-servant-leadership. Accessed October 10, 2018.

14. Walker J. A new call to stewardship and servant leadership. *Nonprofit World*. 2003;21(4):25.

15. Martinuzzi B. *The Leader as a Mensch: How to Become the Kind of Person Others Want to Follow*. Freedom, CA: Six Seconds; 2009.

16. Timmons JA, Spinelli S. *New Venture Creation: Entrepreneurship for the 21st Century*. McGraw-Hill/Irwin; 2007.

17. Sandstrom RW. The meanings of autonomy for physical therapy. *Phys Ther*. 2007;87(1):98-106. doi:10.2522/ ptj.20050245

18. Swisher LL, Page CG. *Professionalism in Physical Therapy: History, Practice & Development*. St. Louis, MO: Elsevier Saunders; 2005.

19. Covey SMR. *The SPEED of TRUST: The One Thing That Changes Everything*. New York, NY: Simon & Schuster; 2006.

20. Lowney C. *Heroic Leadership: Best Practices from a 450-Year-Old Company That Changed the World*. Chicago, IL: Loyola Press; 2009.

21. Ganz M. Leading change: Leadership, organization, and social movements. *Handb Leadersh Theory Pract*. 2010;19.

Suggested Readings

Bolman LG, Deal TE. *Leading With Soul*. 3rd ed. San Francisco, CA: John Wiley & Sons; 2011.

Covey SMR. *The SPEED of TRUST*. New York, NY: Free Press; 2006.

Financial Disclosures

Dr. Eileen C. Bach has no financial or proprietary interest in the materials presented herein.

Dr. Janet R. Bezner has no financial or proprietary interest in the materials presented herein.

Dr. Jill Black has no financial or proprietary interest in the materials presented herein.

Dr. Diane E. Clark has no financial or proprietary interest in the materials presented herein.

Beth Danehy has no financial or proprietary interest in the materials presented herein.

Dr. Joshua D'Angelo has no financial or proprietary interest in the materials presented herein.

Dr. Jennifer Green-Wilson has no financial or proprietary interest in the materials presented herein.

Dr. Efosa L. Guobadia has no financial or proprietary interest in the materials presented herein.

Karen M. Hughes has no financial or proprietary interest in the materials presented herein.

Richard Jackson has no financial or proprietary interest in the materials presented herein.

Dr. Geneva Richard Johnson has no financial or proprietary interest in the materials presented herein.

Dr. Nancy R. Kirsch has no financial or proprietary interest in the materials presented herein.

Craig Moore has no financial or proprietary interest in the materials presented herein.

Dr. Karen Mueller has no financial or proprietary interest in the materials presented herein.

Dr. Sheila K. Nicholson has no financial or proprietary interest in the materials presented herein.

Angela M. Phillips has no financial or proprietary interest in the materials presented herein.

Dr. Emma K. Stokes has no financial or proprietary interest in the materials presented herein.

Dr. Laura Lee (Dolly) Swisher has no financial or proprietary interest in the materials presented herein.

Dr. Barbara A. Tschoepe has no financial or proprietary interest in the materials presented herein.

Jerre van den Bent has no financial or proprietary interest in the materials presented herein.

Beth Whitehead has no financial or proprietary interest in the materials presented herein.

Dr. Stacey Zeigler has no financial or proprietary interest in the materials presented herein.

Index

Printed in the United States
by Baker & Taylor Publisher Services